Folk Remedies From HAWAI'I

By Ann Kondo Corum

BESS PRESS, INC.
BOX 22388
HONOLULU, HI 96822

To Van E. for encouraging me to be myself
and
To Ken for the inspiration that changed my life.

Library of Congress Catalog Card Number: 86-70672
Corum, Ann Kondo
  Folk Remedies from Hawai'i
Honolulu, Hawaii: Bess Press, Inc.
144 pages

ISBN: 0-935848-37-1
Copyright © 1985 by Ann Kondo Corum
ALL RIGHTS RESERVED
Printed in the United States of America

Cover: Ann Kondo Corum
Design: Ann Corum and Ann Rayson
Typesetting: Stats 'n Graphics
Technical Assistance: Steve Shiraki
Cover Photo: Tony Anjo

CONTENTS

Preface	iv
Childbirth, Children and Convalescence	1
Aches and Pains	15
Bites, Stings, and Other Skin Things	29
Burns, Wounds, and Sores	45
Coughs, Colds, and Fever	57
Head Stuff	77
Stomach Problems	91
Other Pilikia	103
A Short Glossary of Remedies	117
Readings	137

Preface

This book is an offspring of *Folk Wisdom From Hawai'i*. As I collected bits of wisdom for that book, I noticed that many fell into the category of folk remedies. Talking to local folk, I realized that there was a wealth of information in this area. Even the most sophisticated of us believe in magic, and much magic has to do with medicine and medical advice. Known as old wives' tales, home cures, or folk remedies, these treatments are sometimes looked down upon, but most of us are not one hundred percent convinced that there isn't some truth to these home cures. In fact, many prescription drugs have a foundation in natural medicines, and many natural health remedies do indeed have curative powers.

Like all primitive people, the ancient Hawaiians learned which plants cured certain ailments. But they also had a class of medical practitioners, a special kind of kahuna called kahuna lā'au lapa'au, who were trained to prescribe herbal medicines.

When the Europeans began to arrive in Hawai'i, they brought with them new diseases. They also brought with them plants such as aloe, garlic, onion, and tobacco which were quickly adopted and assimilated by the kahuna lā'au lapa'au for use in medical treatment. Later, Orientals who came as plantation laborers brought with them medical lore from their own lands. So like other aspects of Hawai'i's culture, its medical folklore is a rich blend. Folk medicine in Hawai'i today consists of fragments of treatment from kahuna lā'au lapa'au as well as treatment from Orientals and Caucasians. It is interesting to note that many distant cultures have similar cures.

The first section of the book relates remedies for ailments by subject. Sometimes an explanation is given. Like folk wisdom, folk remedies are often passed down from generation to generation as "tribal truth." One can accept these bits of wisdom, totally discredit them, or believe some and not others. Unlike previously published books on medicinal herbs and folk medicine in Hawai'i, this book is meant to be a popular rather than a scholarly treatment of things of medicinal value. It is also an attempt to list remedies in an accessible way. In the second part of the book, I have attempted to include a descriptive section on some plants and other things used in folk remedies. This is only a very brief cross section of some frequently recurring items.

The book is addressed to the general reader and in no way attempts to include self-treatment of serious diseases. Simple remedies such as the ones listed may be beneficial for uncomplicated illnesses or basic first aid. However, a physician should be consulted for more serious illnesses. My aim is to introduce some of Hawai'i's medical folklore in an entertaining fashion and from a sociological perspective. In no way do I intend to prescribe treatment of any kind.

When using any folk remedy, one should take sensible precautions. Some points to keep in mind include:
- Do not use plants that are unidentified.
- Do not use plants that are narcotic.
- Don't take several remedies at one time.
- Take any remedy in moderation.
- See a doctor if a condition persists.

While I have not cited specific references in the text, a bibliography is appended for those of you who may want to read more on the subject. Thanks go out to all who contributed their remedies to the book. I especially appreciate the contributions from the senior citizens of Hawai'i who, by remembering the past, help to preserve our culture for future generations.

Ann Kondo Corum

Childbirth, Children, and Convalescence

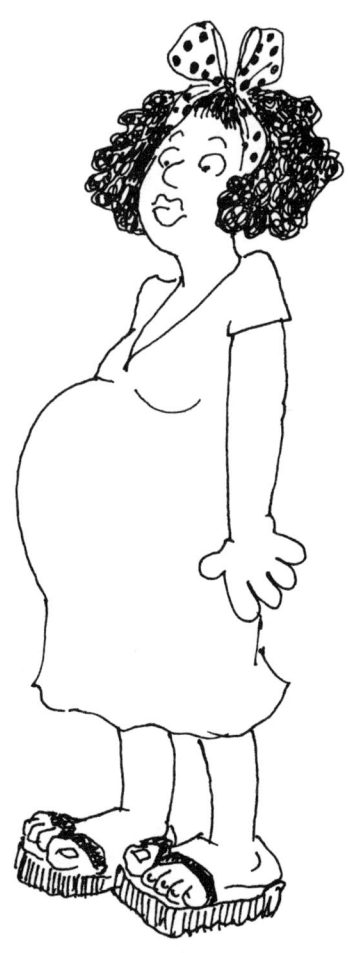

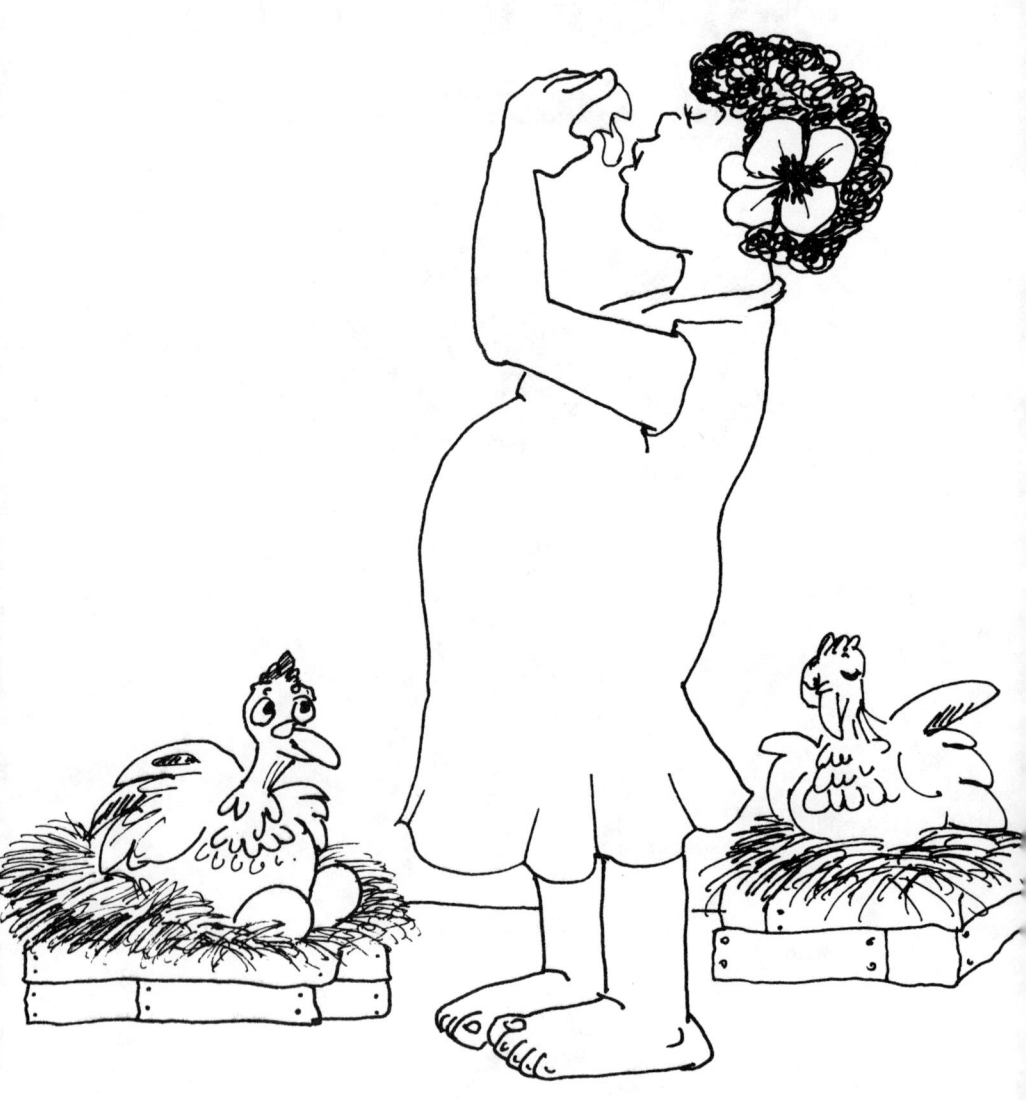

If a pregnant woman eats raw eggs she will have an easy delivery.

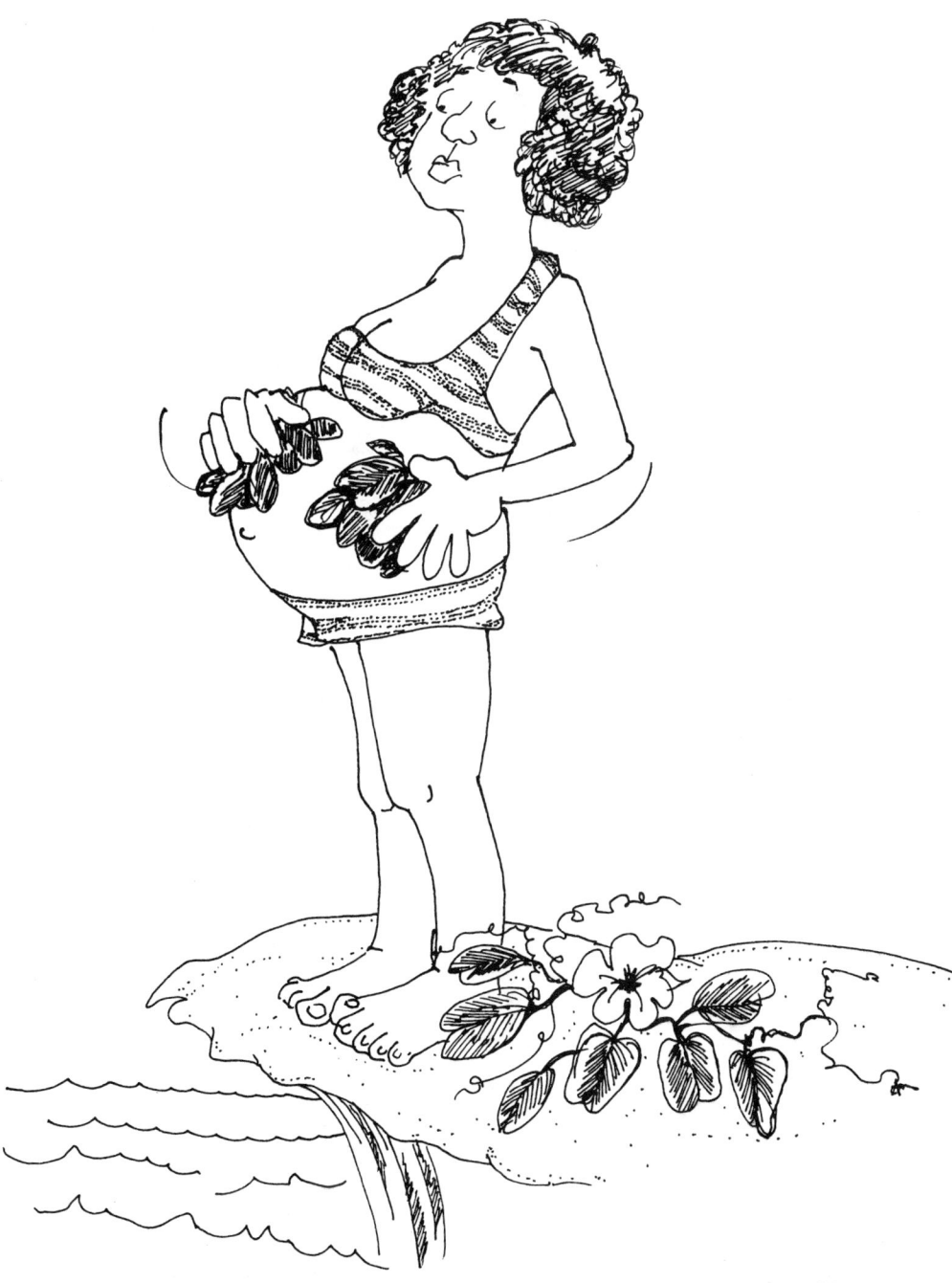

A pregnant woman who wants to hasten the birth of her baby should rub pōhuehue (beach morning glory) on her ʻōpū.

To ease the pains of childbirth, scrape the slimy inside of the bark of the hau tree, mix it with water, and give it to the mother between labor pains.

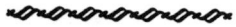

Pregnant women should drink ginseng tonic to ease childbirth and to strengthen the body.

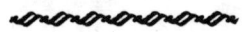

Drink the juice obtained by boiling chrysanthemum leaves for a safe and easy childbirth.

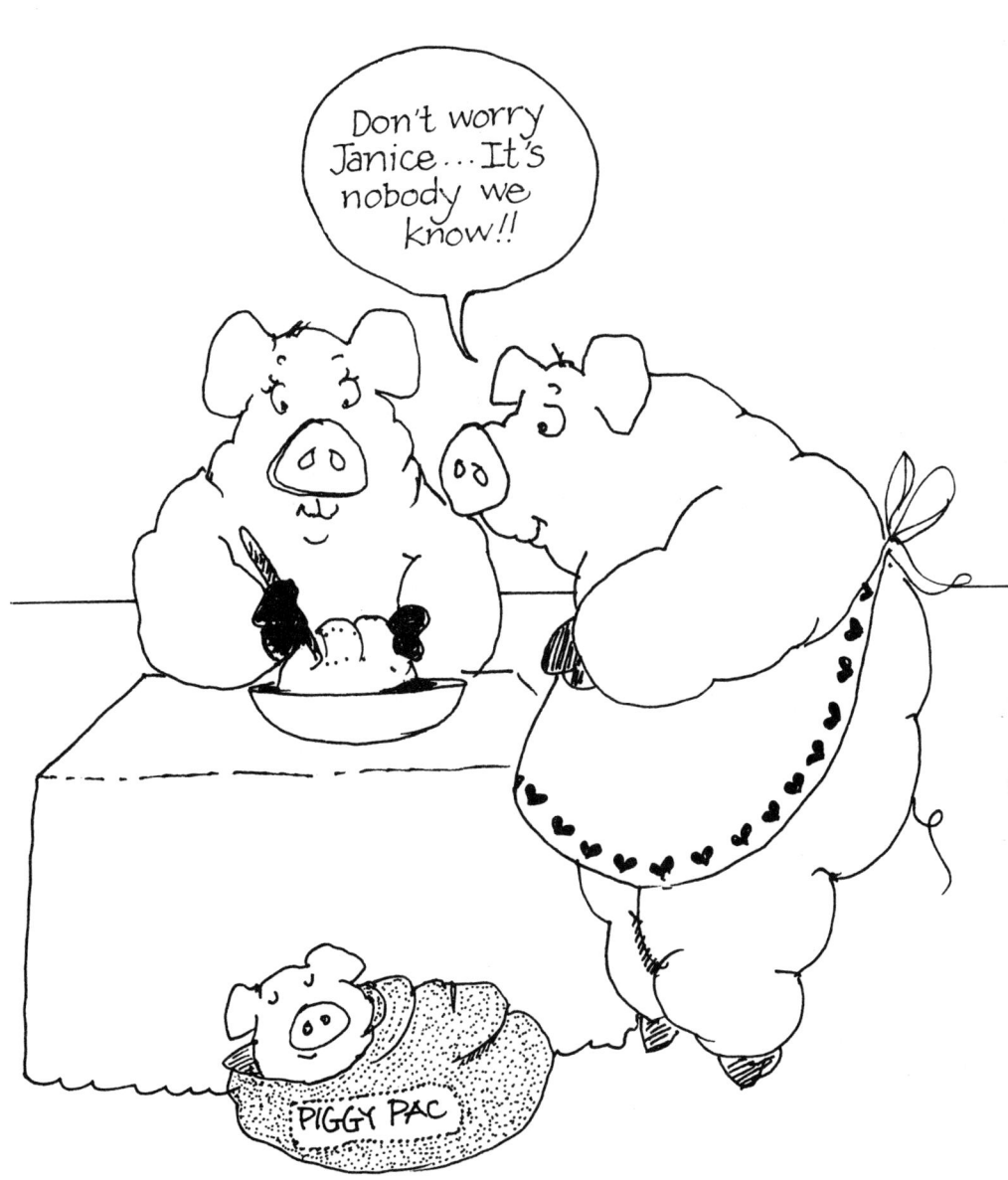

Feed a new mother sweet-sour pigs' feet to increase her milk supply.

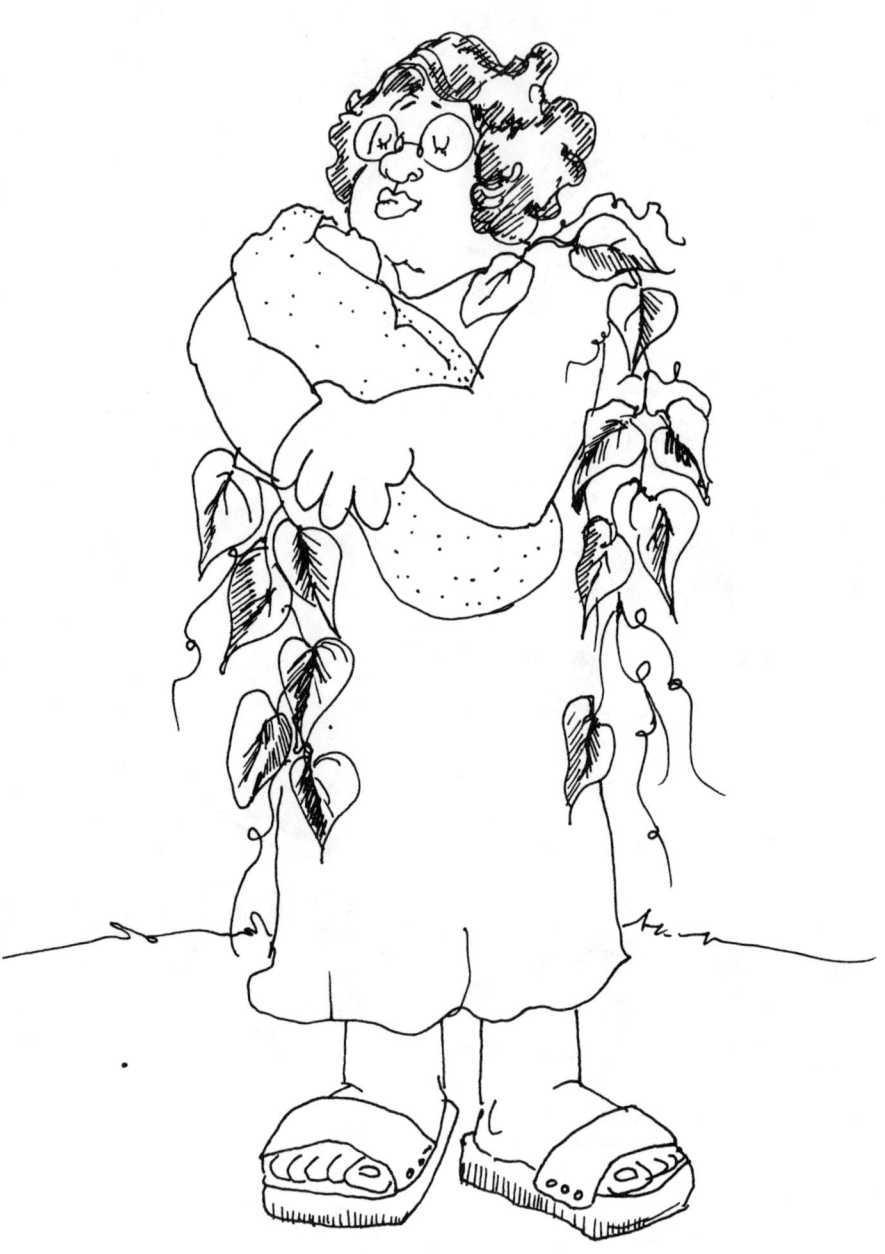

A nursing mother should wear a lei of sweet potato vines around her neck to guarantee a good supply of milk.

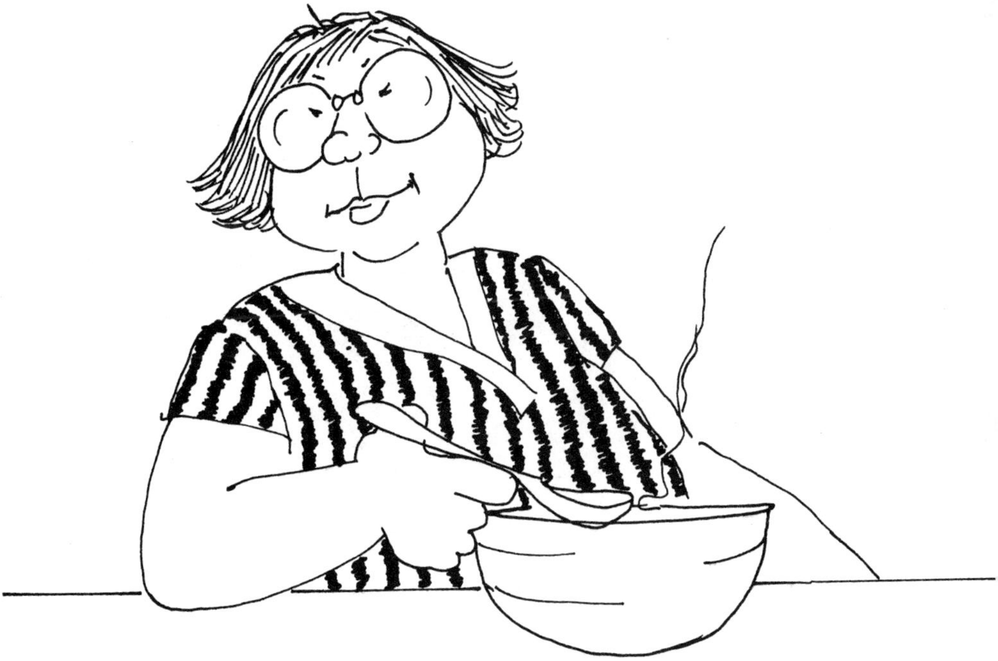

A person convalescing from an illness or a woman recovering from childbirth should eat seaweed soup to regain strength.

After childbirth or a long illness, Chinese eat chicken cooked in liquor and lots of ginger root to strengthen the body and increase one's appetite.

To strengthen a weak baby, Hawaiians chewed limu kala and limu līpoa, mixed it with baked taro, and fed it to the child.

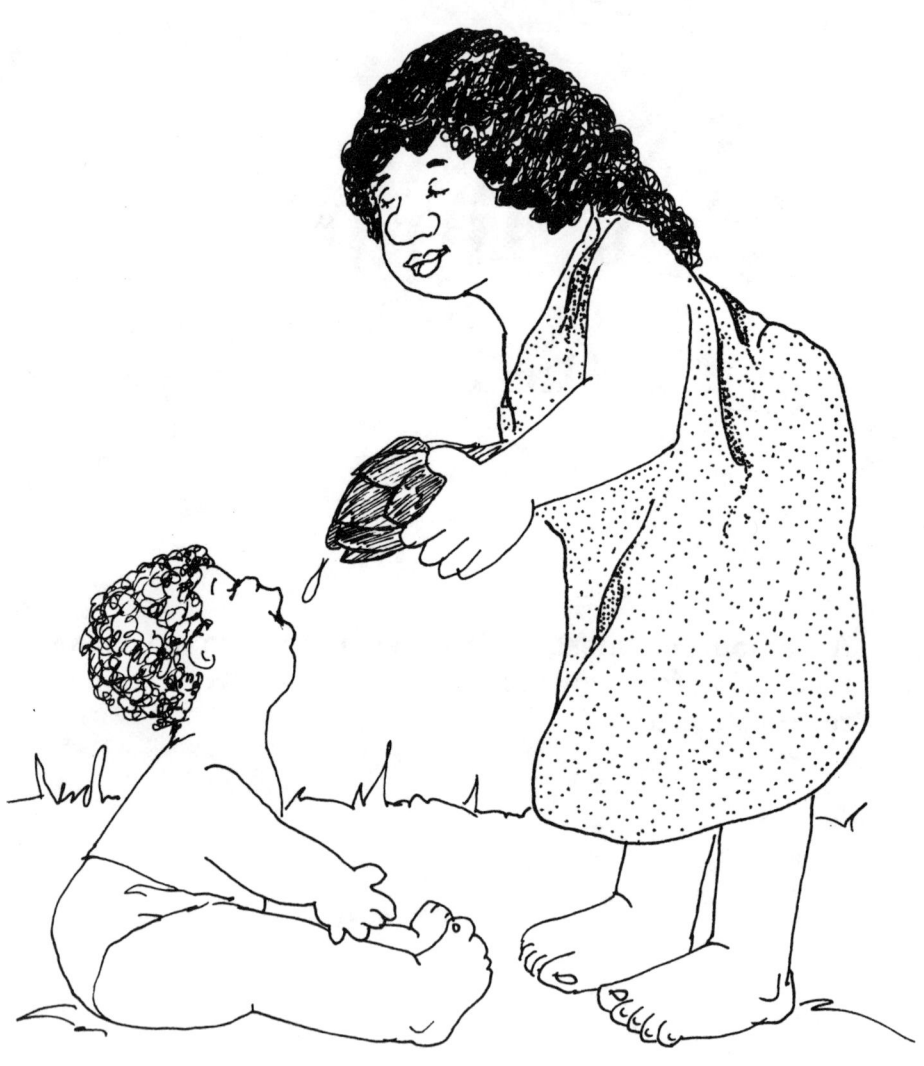

The juice from the tips of banana blossoms was used as a vitamin for babies by ancient Hawaiians.

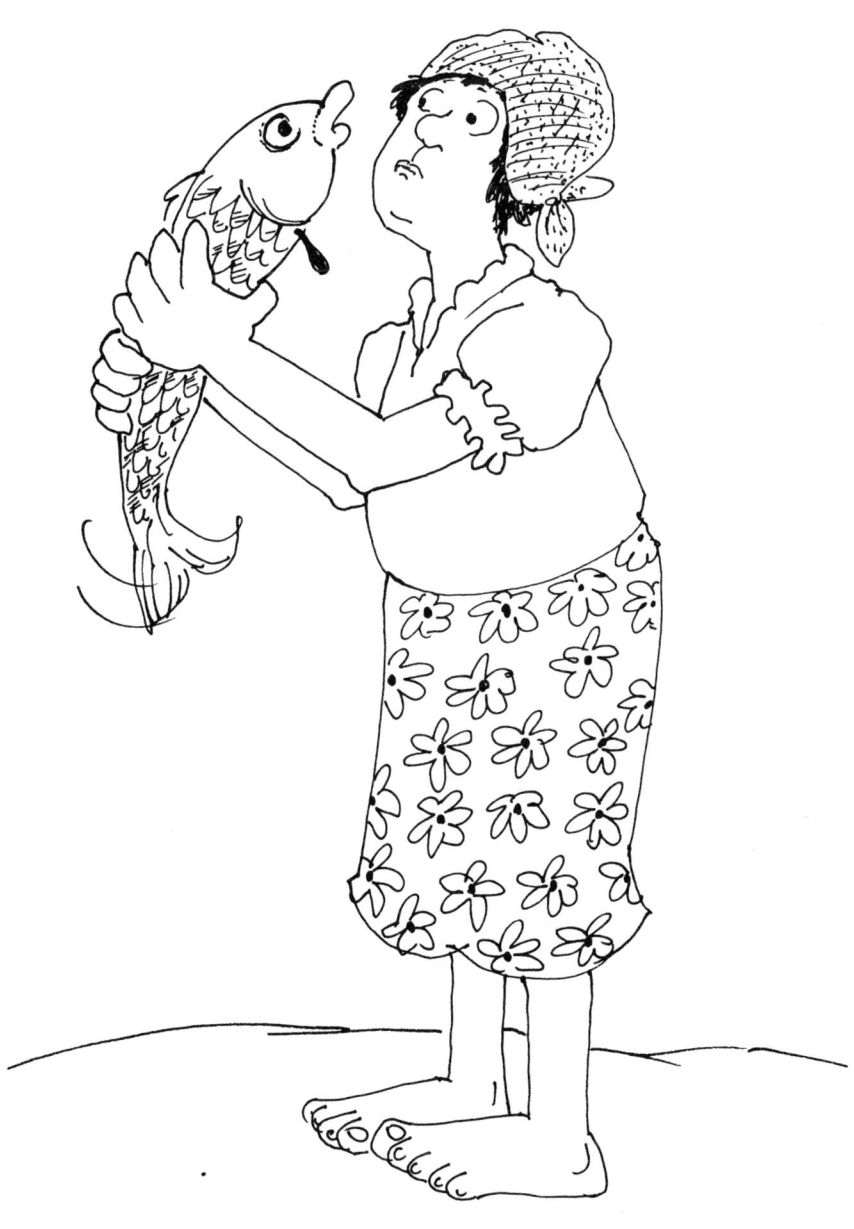

To get rid of a lingering illness, drink the blood of a live carp (make a slit in the fish . . . do not kill it).

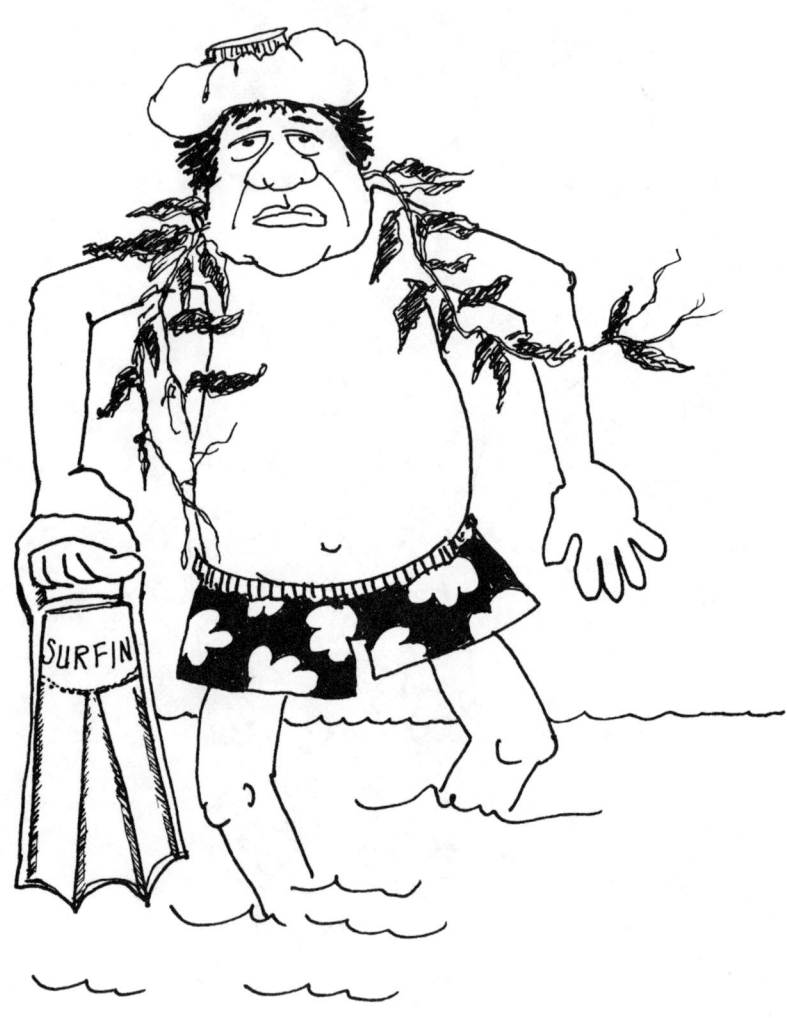

If a person convalescing from an illness wants to be freed from the illness completely, he should make an open lei out of limu kala and swim out to sea with the lei around his neck. The sea washing the lei off his neck washes away the evil causing the illness.

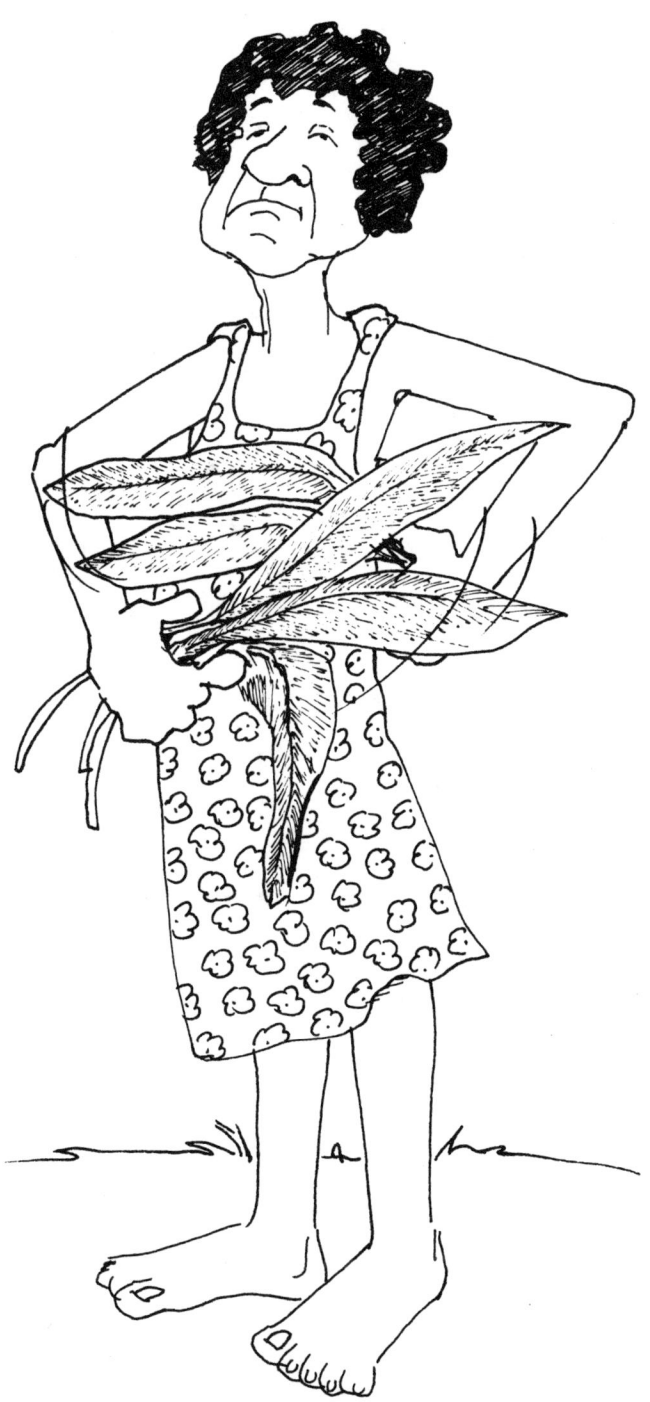

To get rid of an evil spirit causing an illness, slap yourself with a bunch of ti leaves.

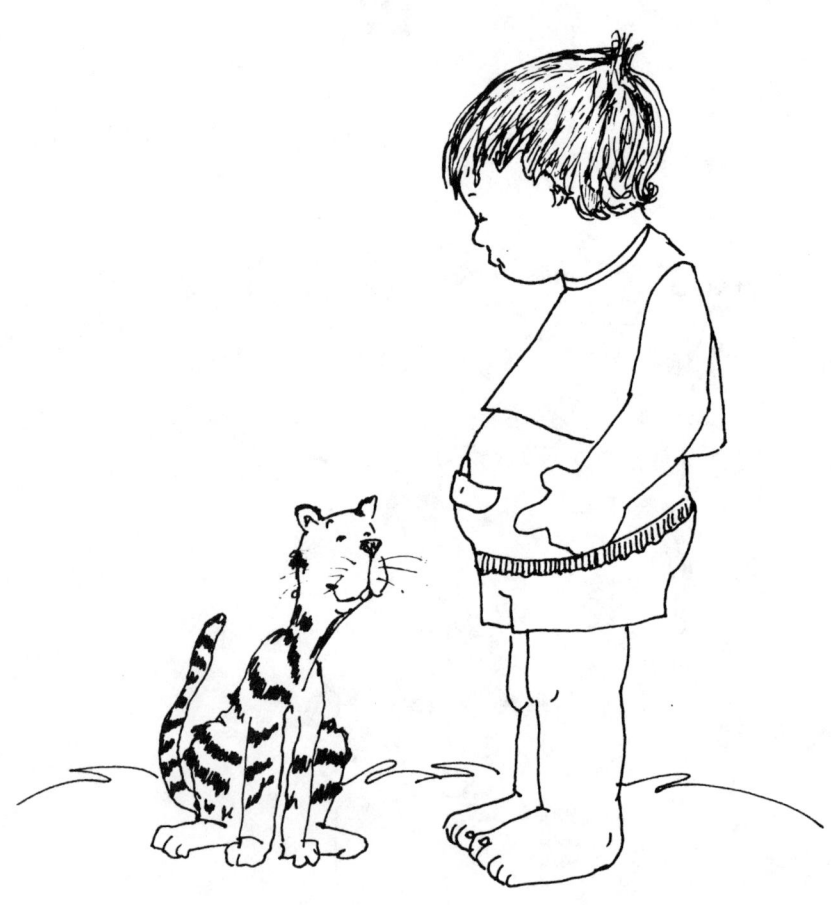

If a baby's belly button pops out, put a coin on it and tape it down to push the belly button in.

Apply yaito to cure bed-wetting in children.

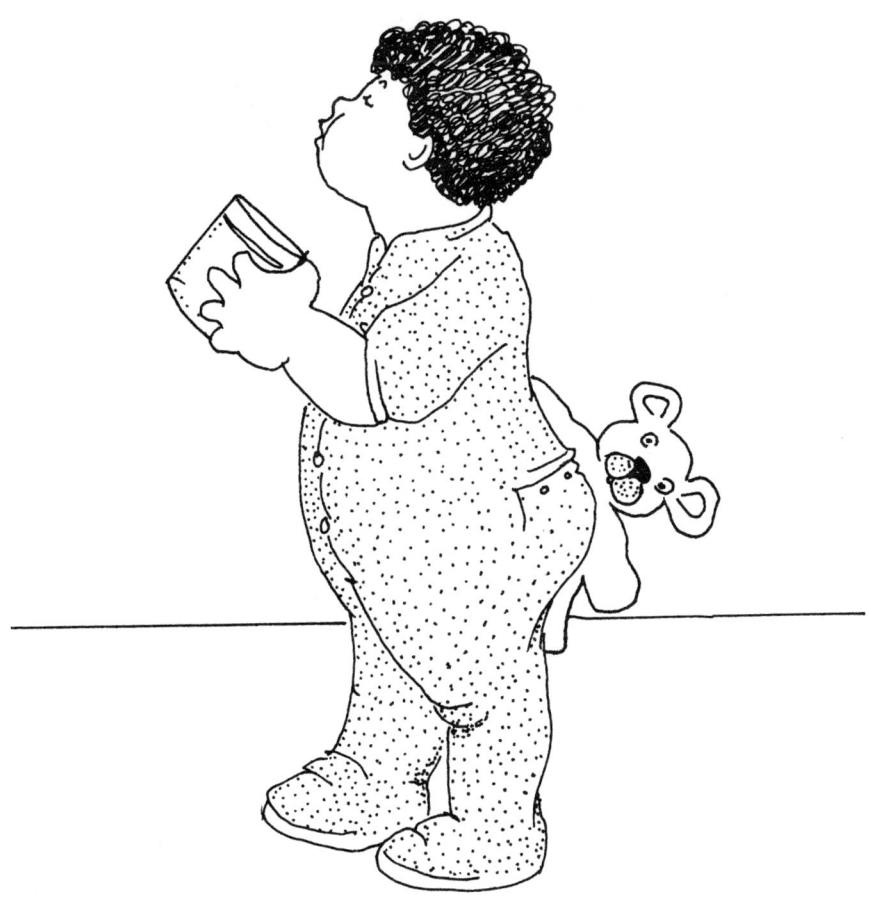

To cure bed-wetting, chew or grind some 'awa root, mash it with a cup of water, and strain the juice. Drink the juice about an hour before going to bed.

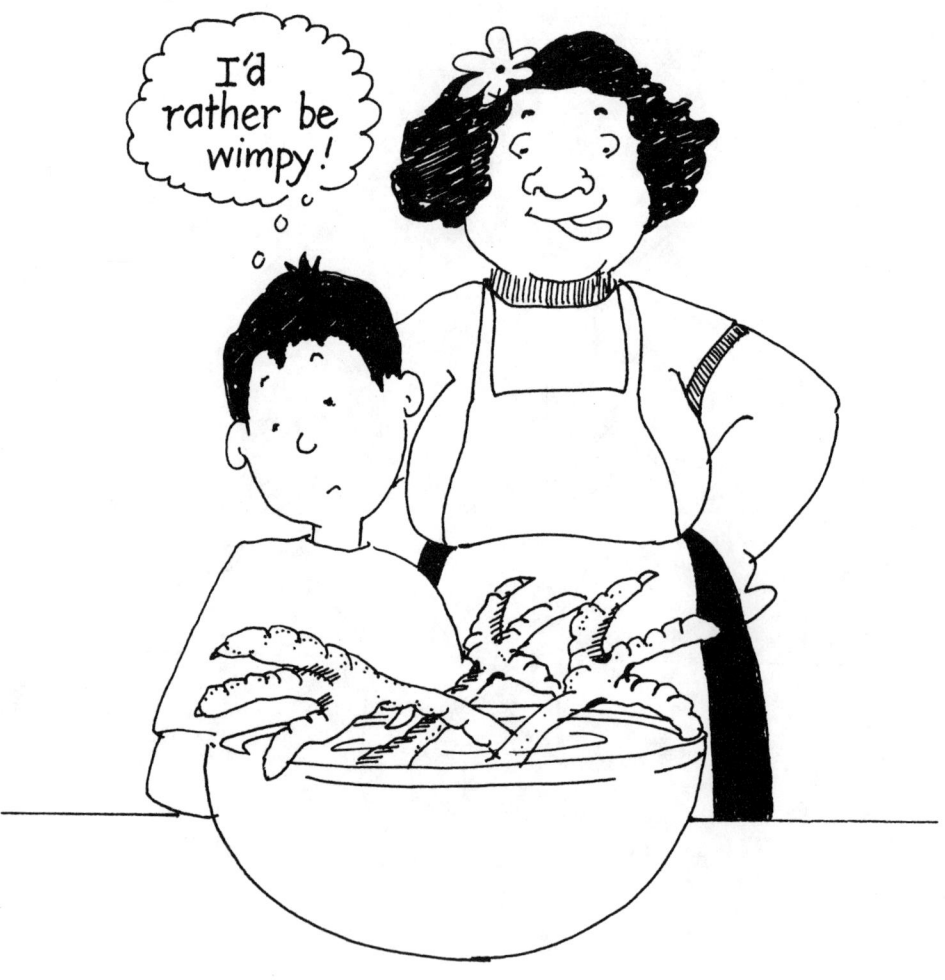

Children who are fed soup made out of chicken feet will develop strong muscles.

Aches and Pains

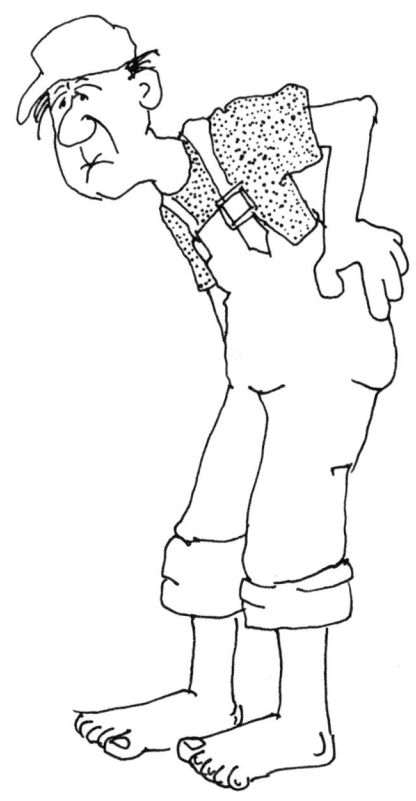

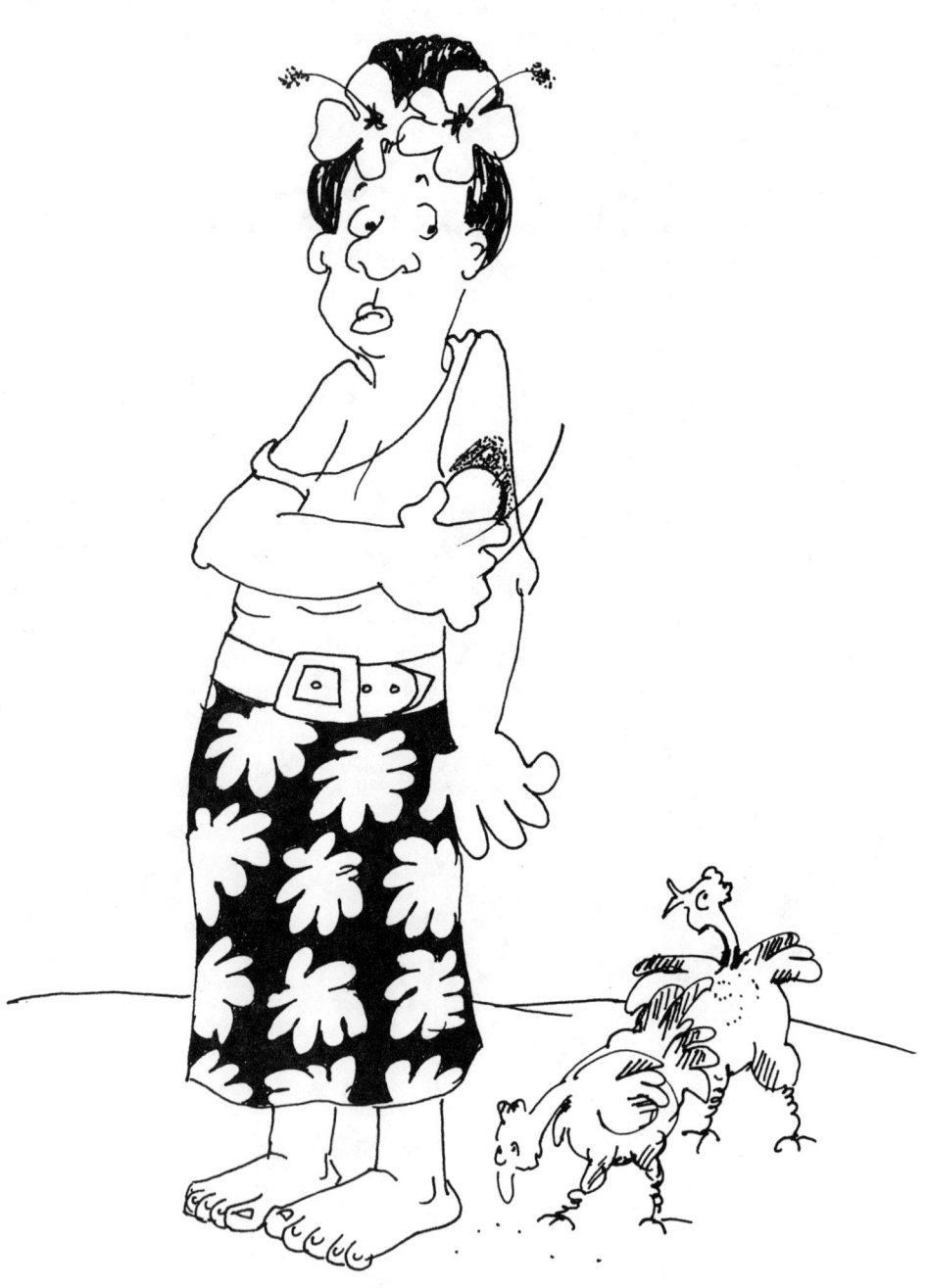

To get rid of a bruise, roll a hard boiled egg on it.

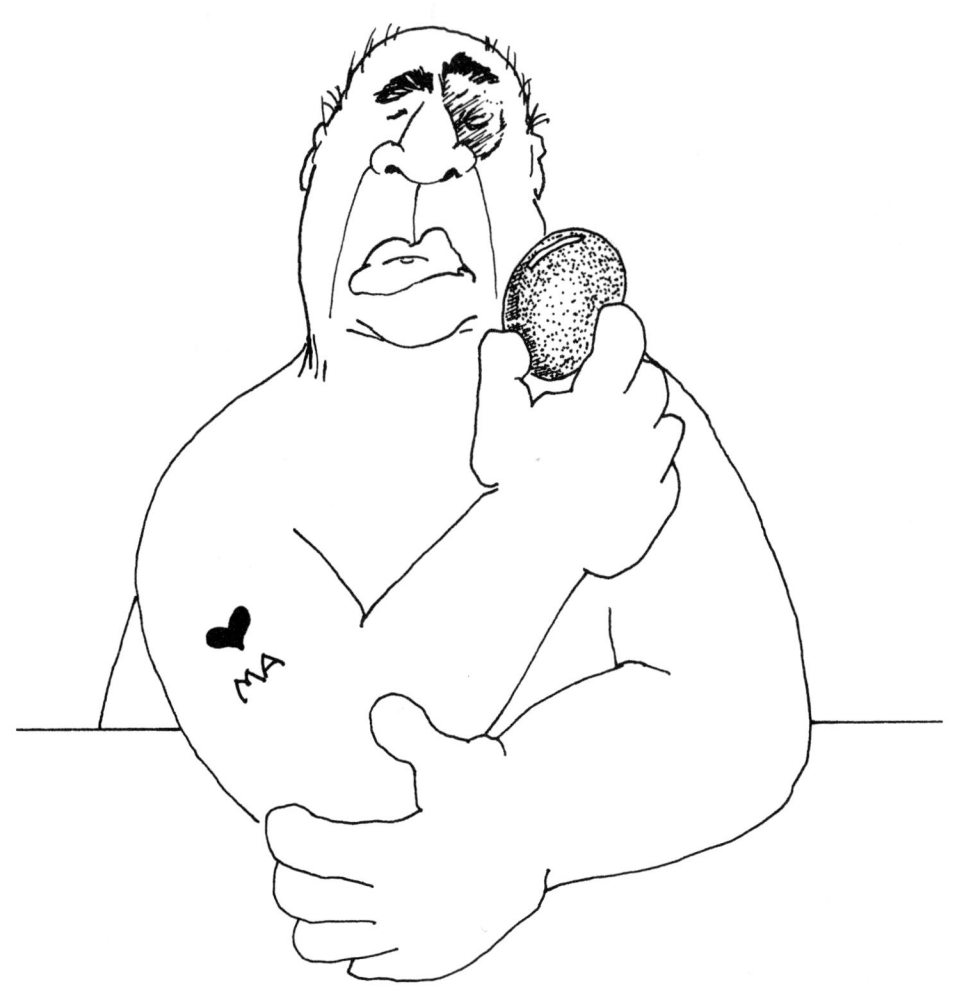

To relieve a black eye, rub a brown egg on it.

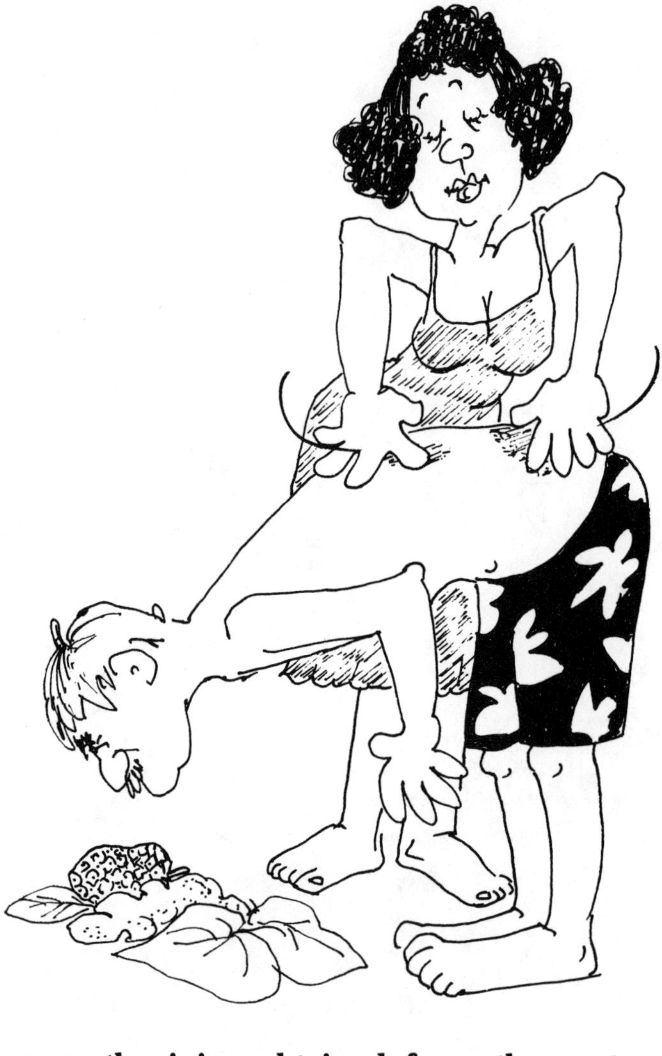

Massage the juice obtained from the roots of wild ginger, 'awa, ripe noni, and a bit of water into sprains and bruises.

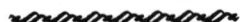

To help bruises heal faster, apply salt water on them.

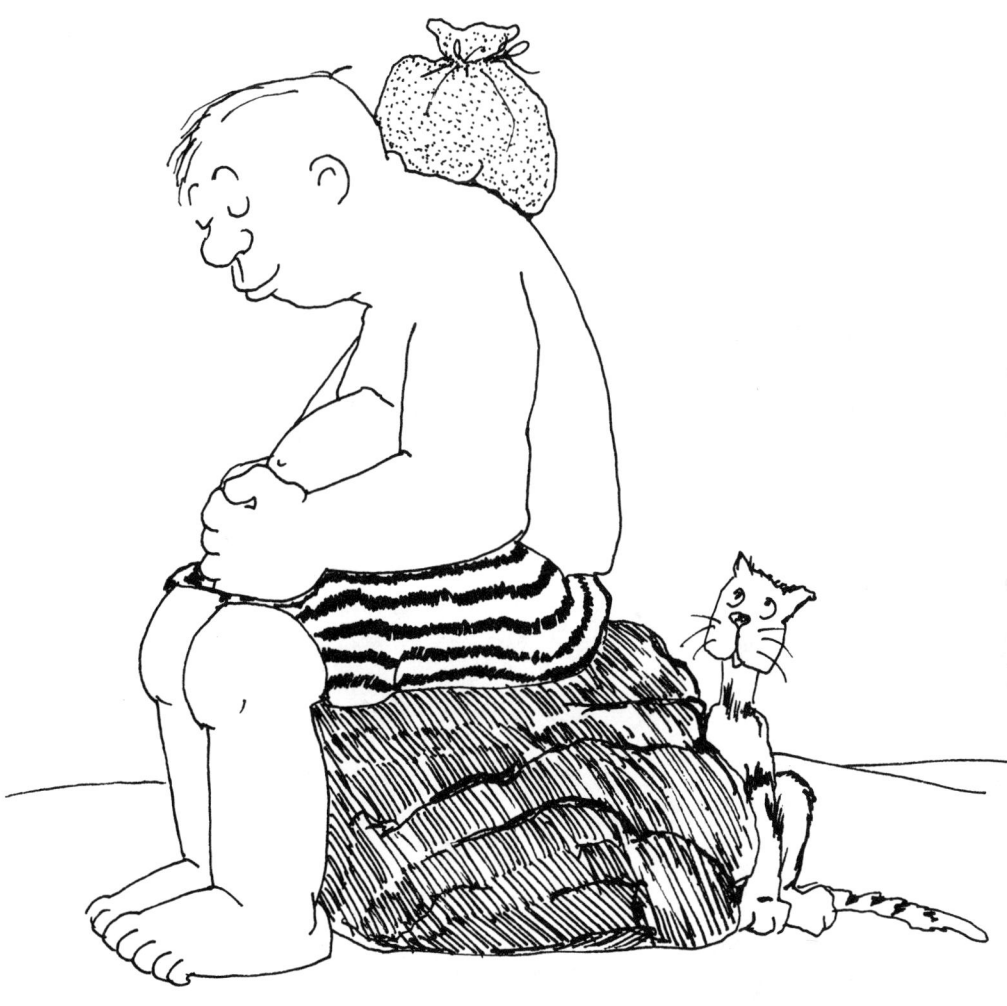

Hawaiian heating pad: Heat Hawaiian salt, put it in a cloth bag, and apply to aches and pains.

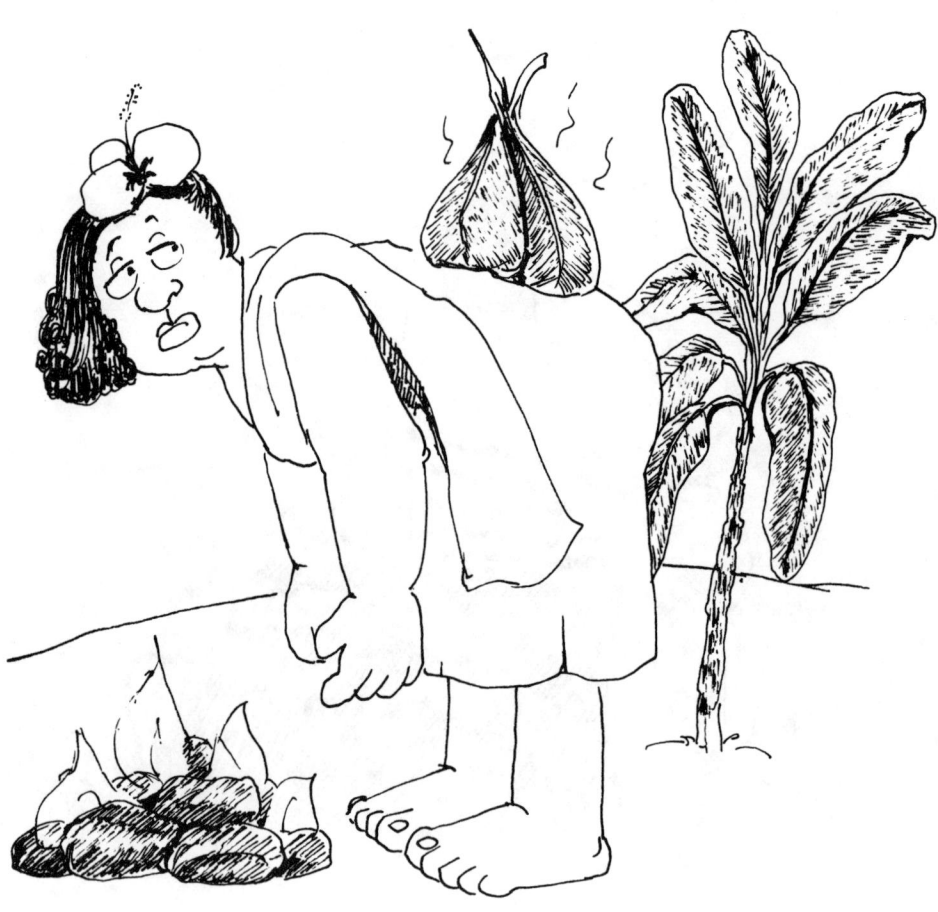

The ancient Hawaiians wrapped hot stones in ti leaves and used them on backaches.

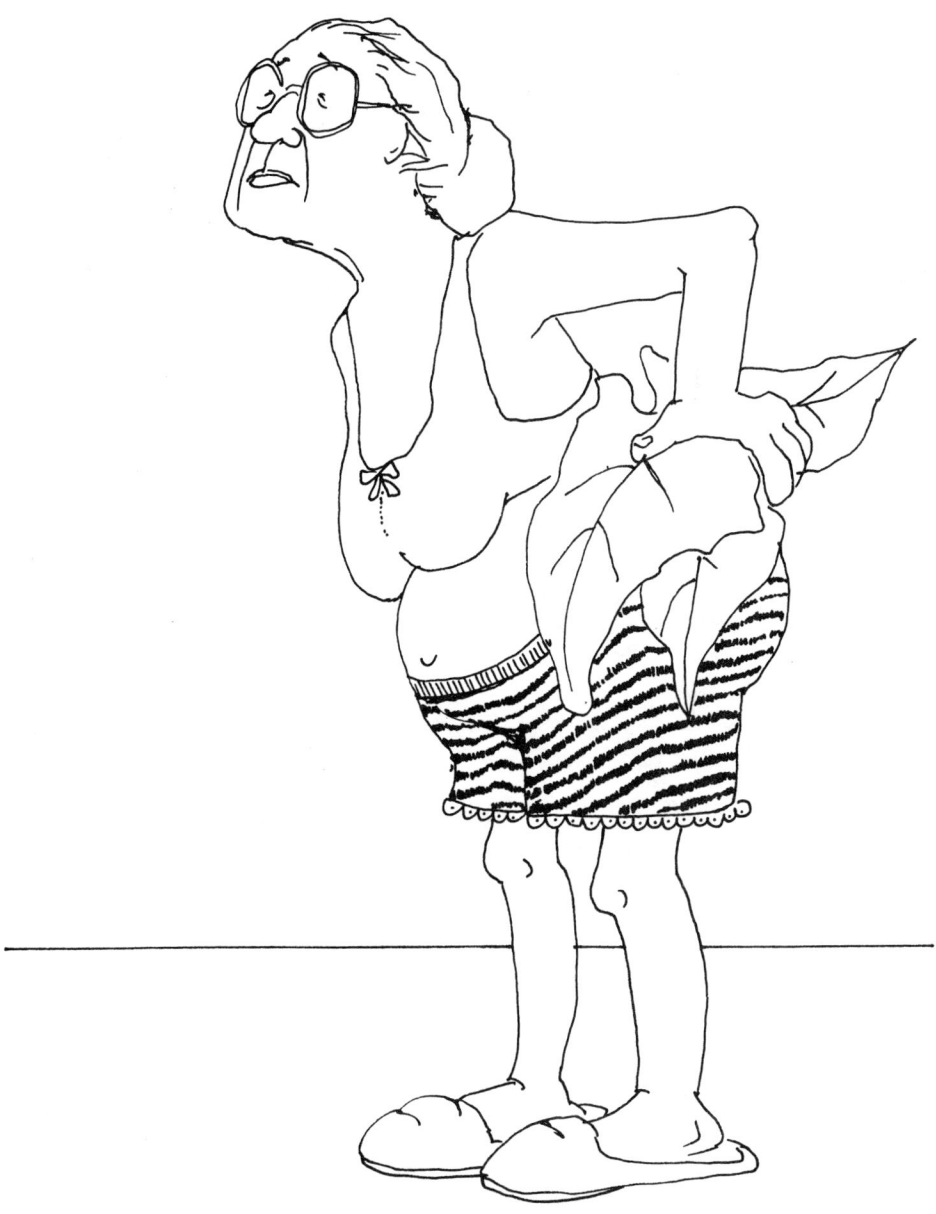

To relieve back pains, bind your back with taro leaves before you go to sleep. Repeat the treatment 4 to 5 nights.

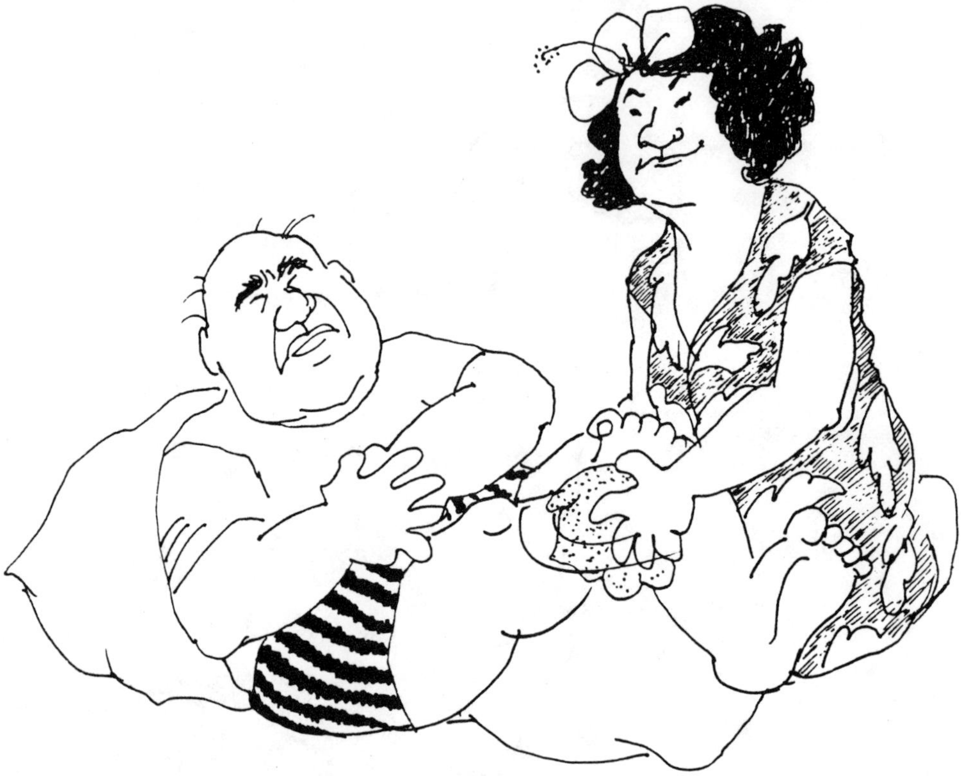

To treat a sprain, cut the top of a sugar cane shoot. Mash it with lots of Hawaiian salt. Wrap it in ti leaves and bake. When it is soft, squeeze out the juice. Saturate a cloth in the juice and rub it on the sprained area.

Make a paste out of flour, egg, and vinegar and apply the mixture on sprains.

Boil the leaves of soursop and apply the liquid on aches and pains.

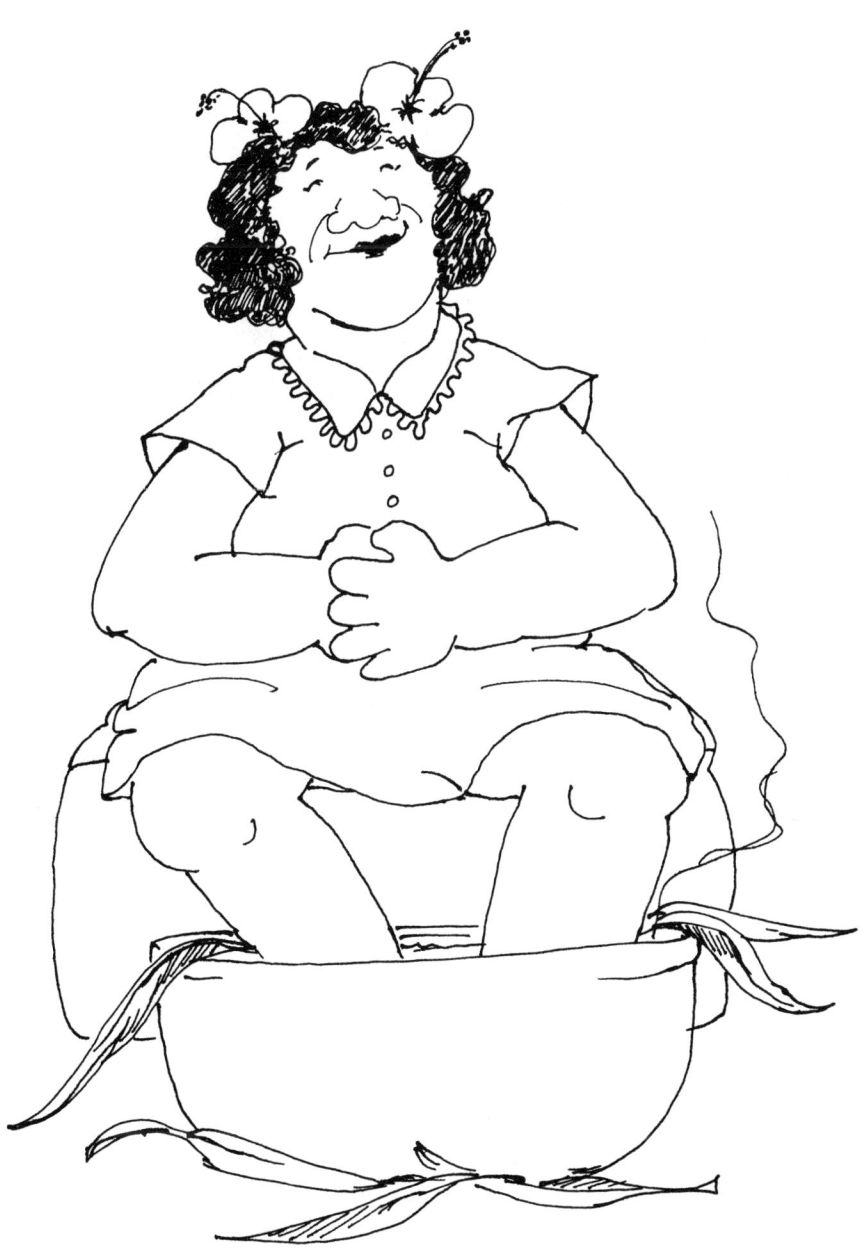

Boil eucalyptus leaves in water and soak sprains in the hot mixture.

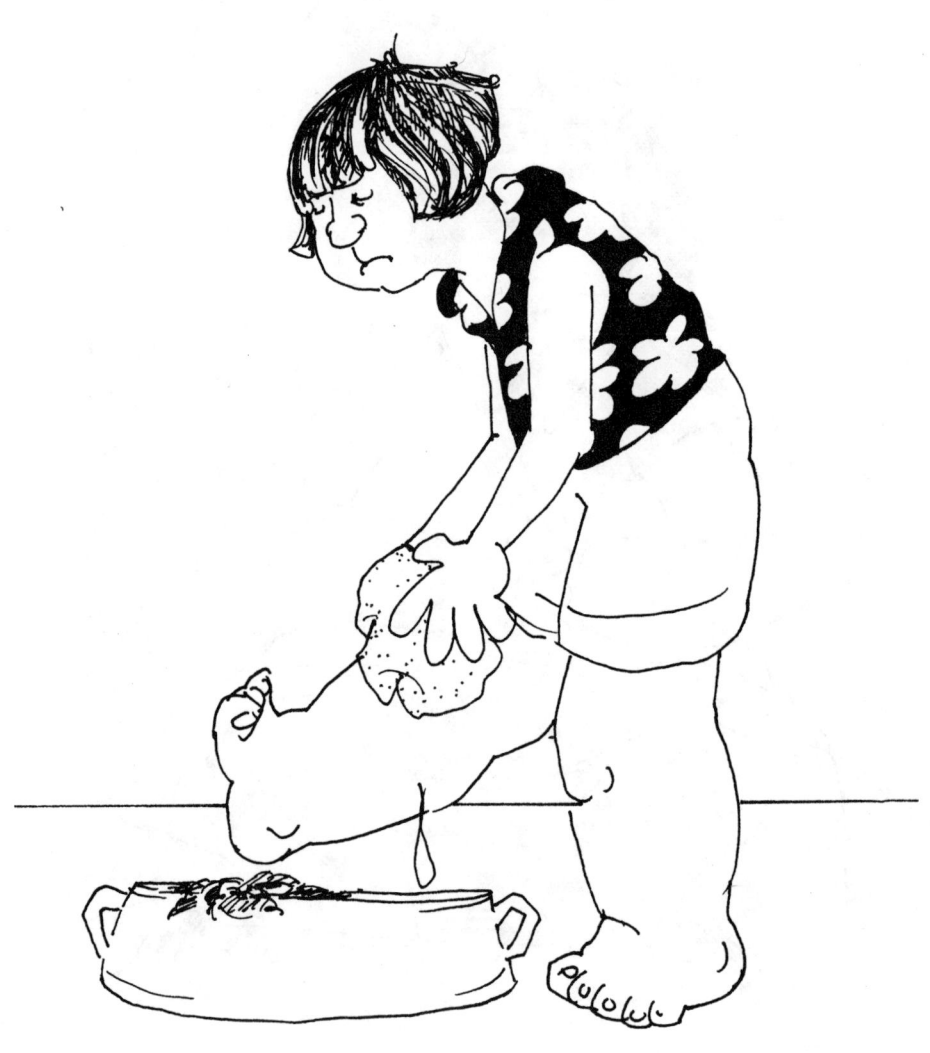

For swollen legs, boil limu and apply the hot water to your legs.

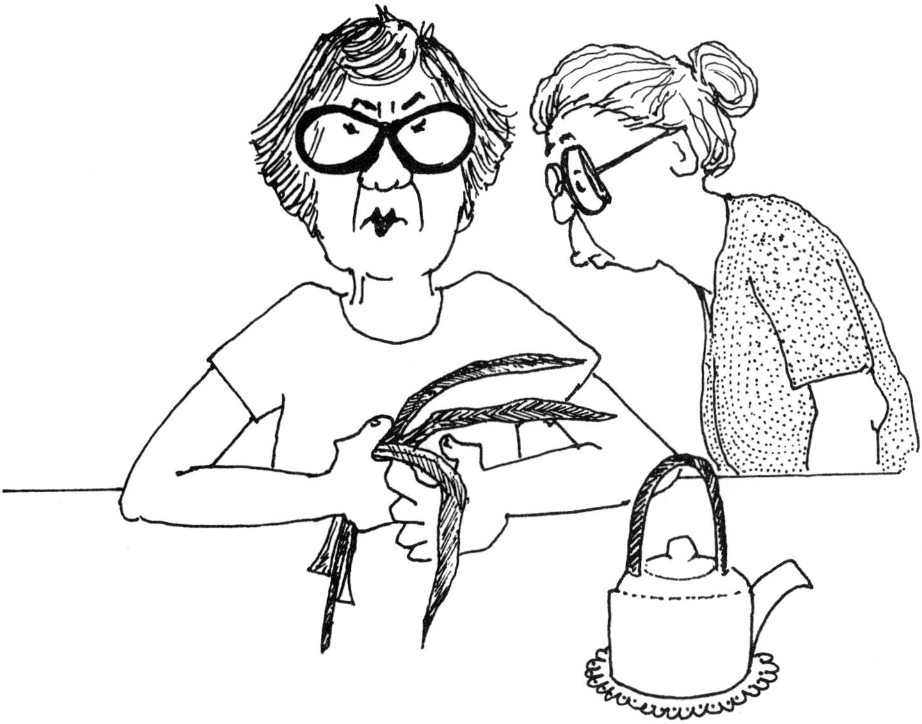

Make a tea out of lemon grass to relieve backache. Take 3 dried leaves, crush them in your hands, and fold them into a small packet. Pour boiling water over them and cover. Drink a cup each morning.

To treat pain due to arthritis, boil some lady slipper flowers in water. Cool the liquid, mix it with wine, and drink it.

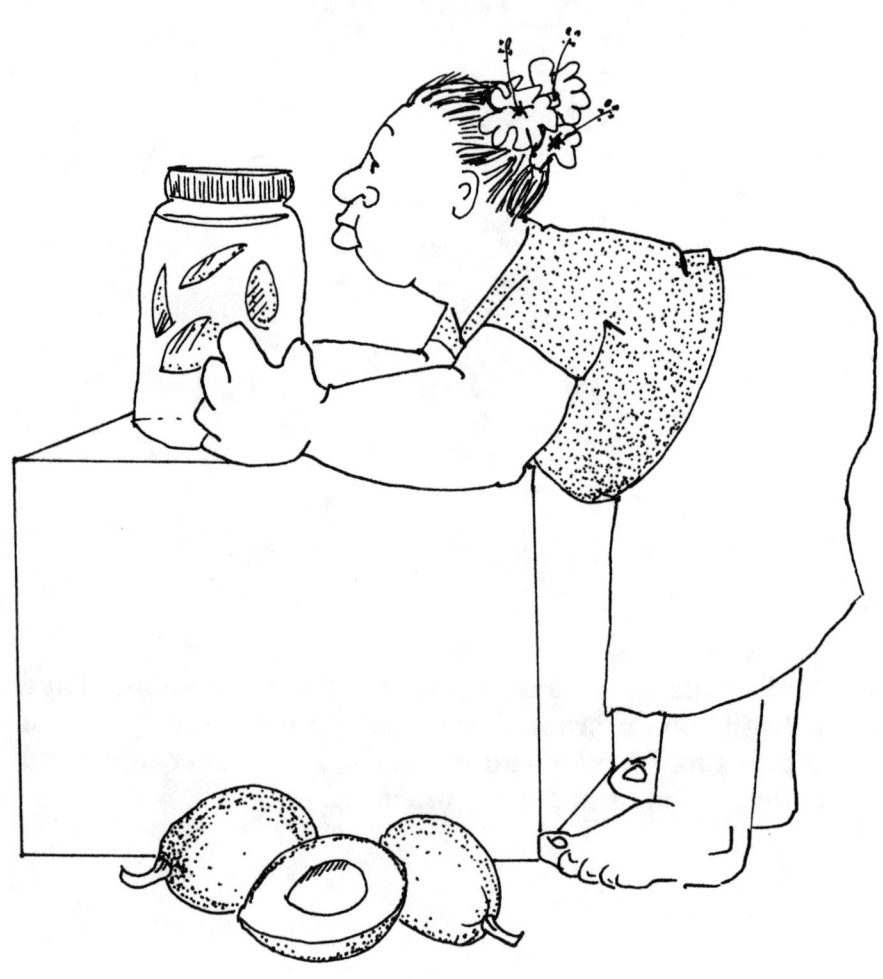

To relieve pain from arthritis, take an avocado seed, chop it into pieces, and put it in a jar with rubbing alcohol. Let it sit 3 to 4 days. Rub the liquid on your aches and pains.

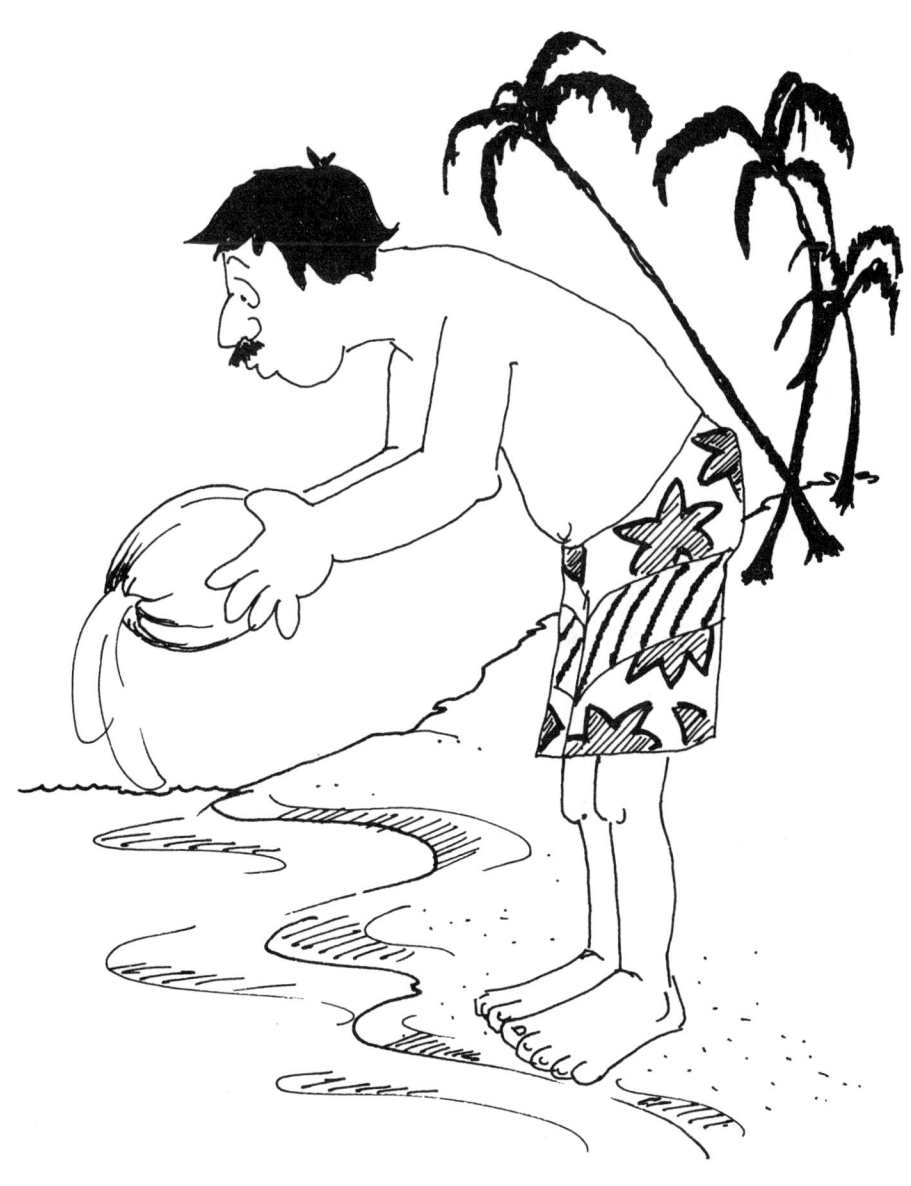

To reduce pain of arthritis, take 1 young coconut, empty the coconut water and replace it with sea water. Let it stand 3 to 4 weeks, then pour out the water and eat the soft coconut.

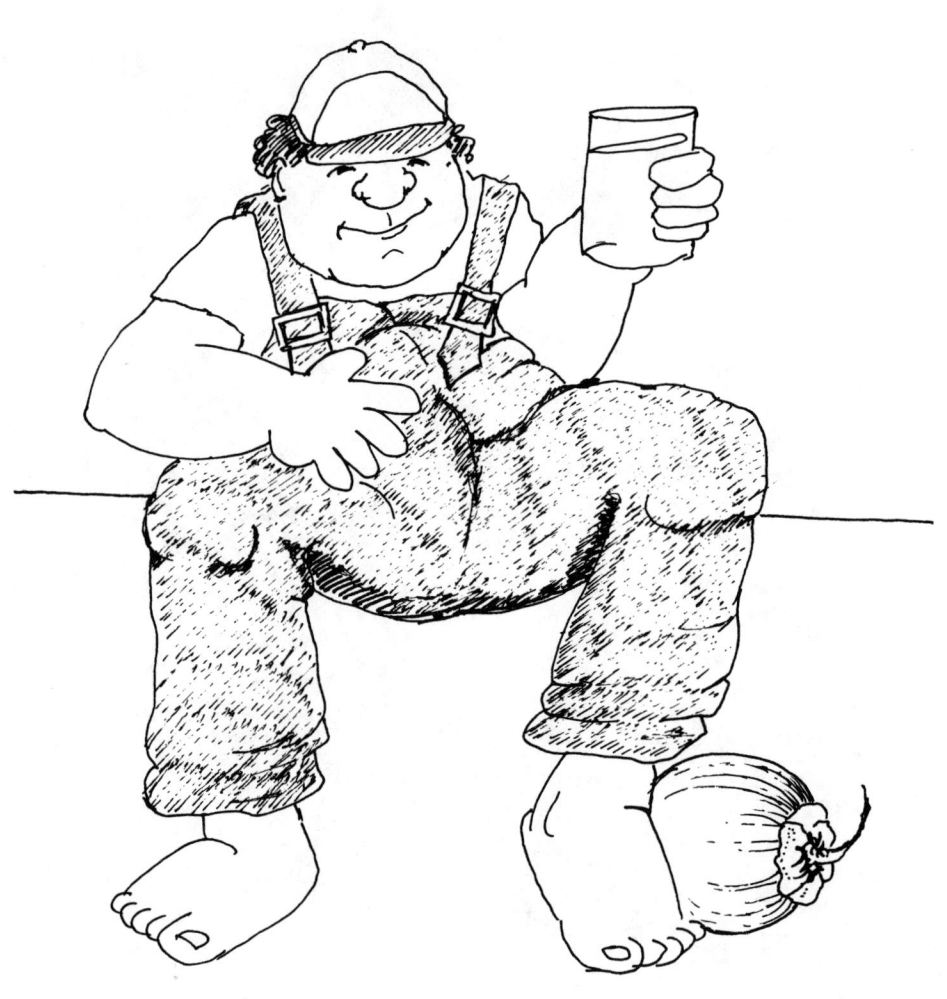

After hard work, drink 'awa mixed with coconut milk to relax muscles and restore strength.

Bites, Stings, and Other Skin Things

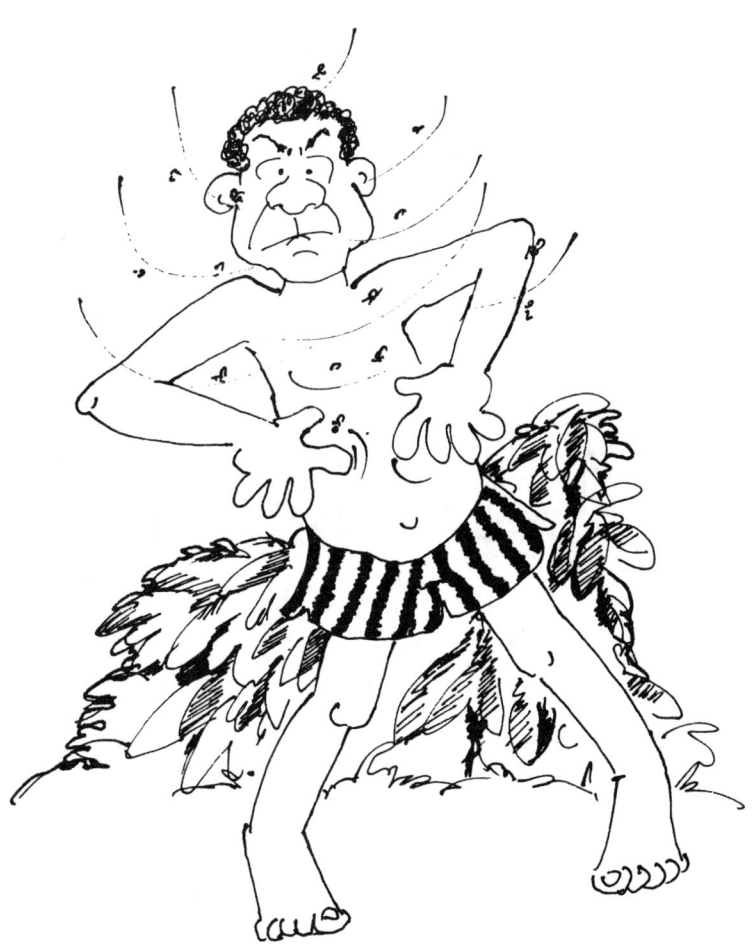

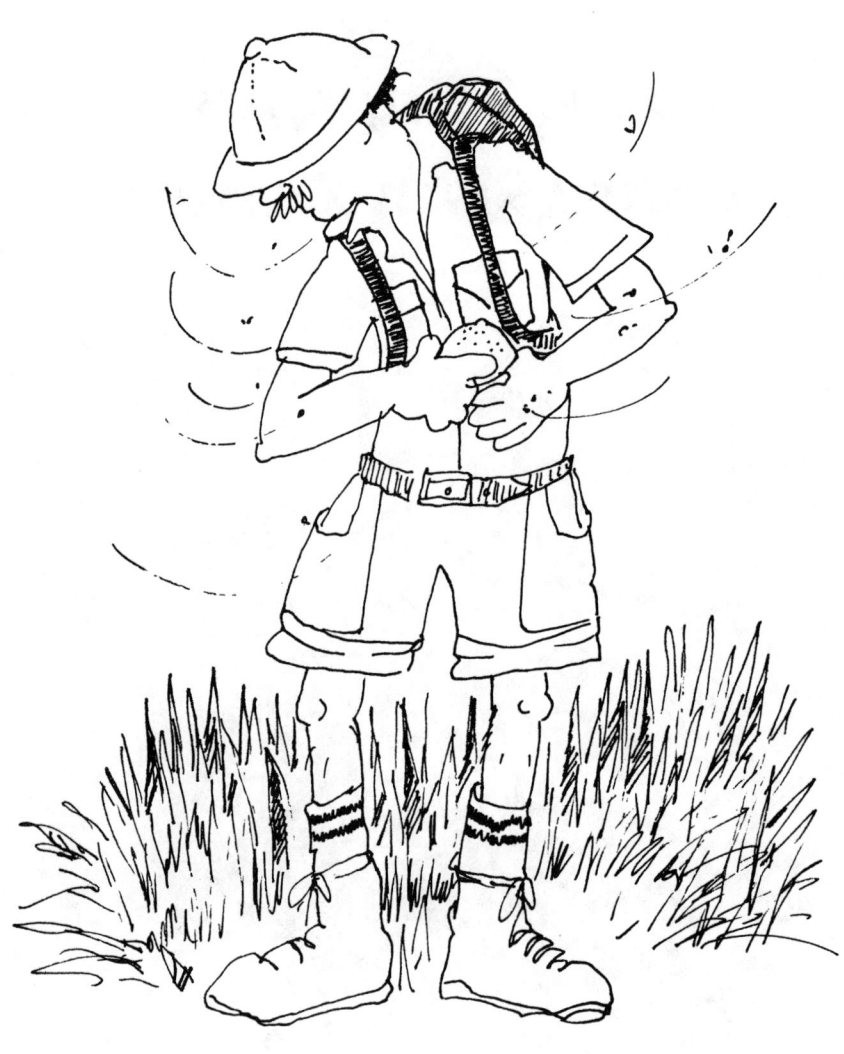

Rub lemon rind on yourself for an effective mosquito repellant.

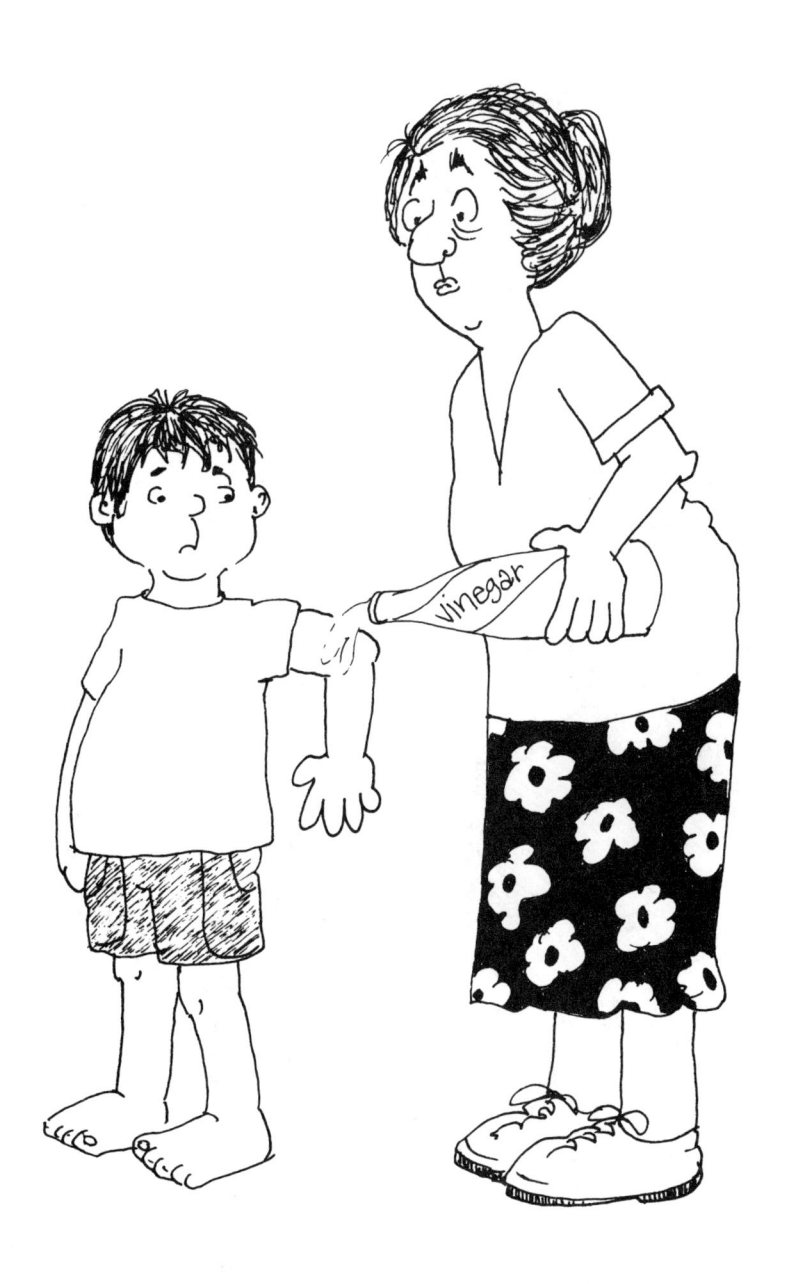

Put vinegar on a bee sting to prevent itching and swelling.

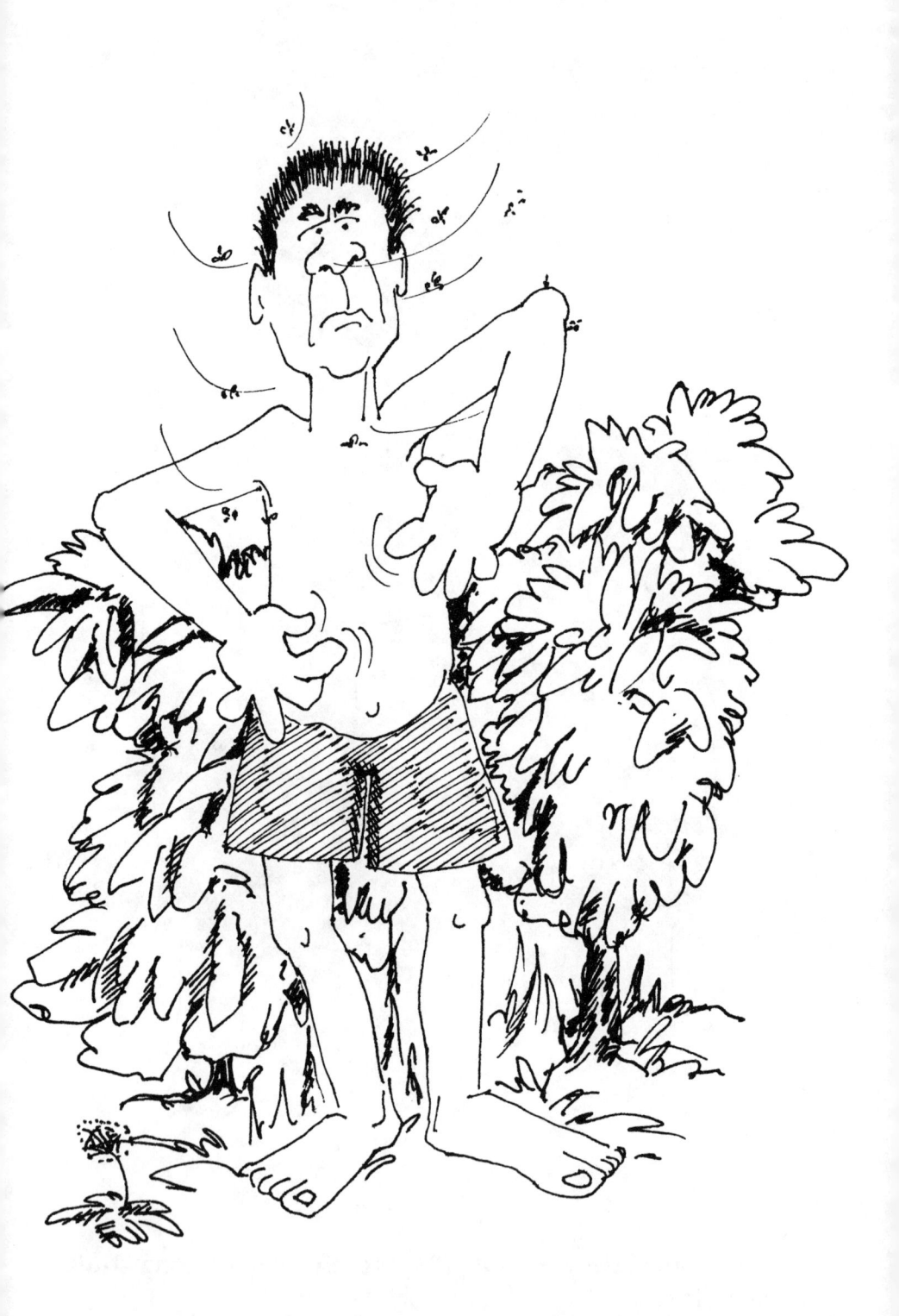

Rub a piece of onion or garlic on insect bites to ease swelling and itching.

To stop pain and itching from insect bites, chew some tea leaves and place them on the affected area.

To reduce swelling from an insect bite, rub a stem of a taro leaf on the bite.

Sores on the skin and rash are quickly healed by the application of mashed dandelion leaves.

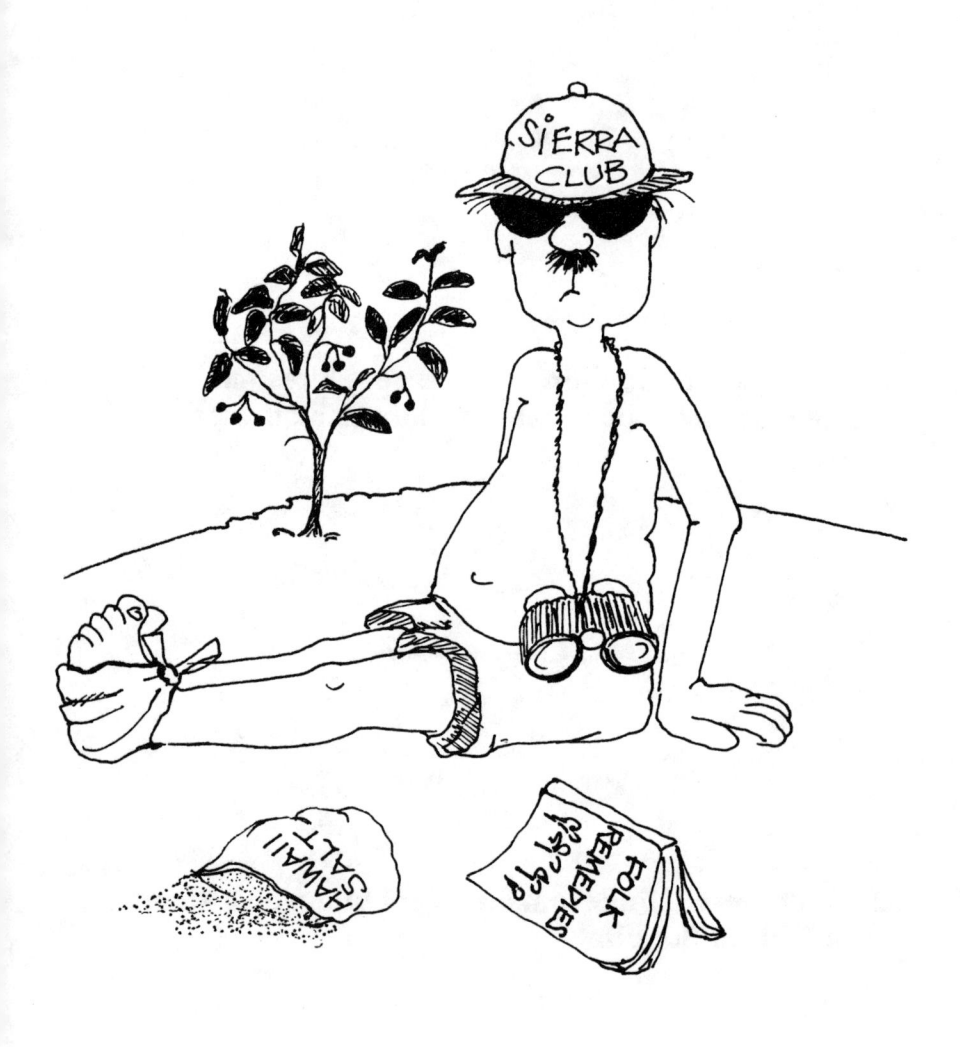

For blisters on the feet and hands, mash some pōpolo leaves with Hawaiian salt, cover the blisters with the mixture, and bind in place with a cloth.

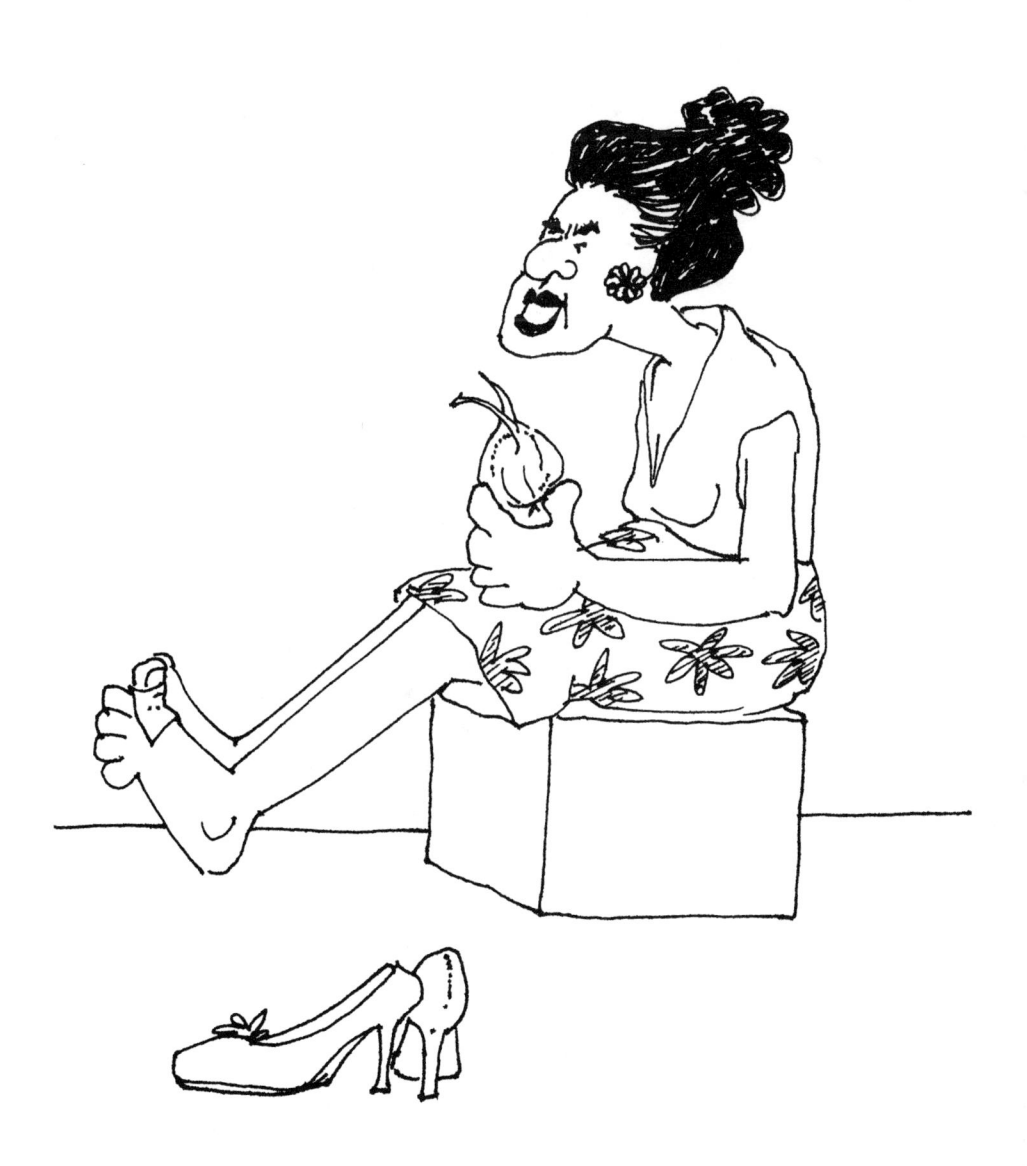

To remove corns from your feet, mash a clove of garlic and the bulbous part of a stalk of green onion. Apply a small amount to the corn and tape it in place. Replace with a fresh application every 2-3 days.

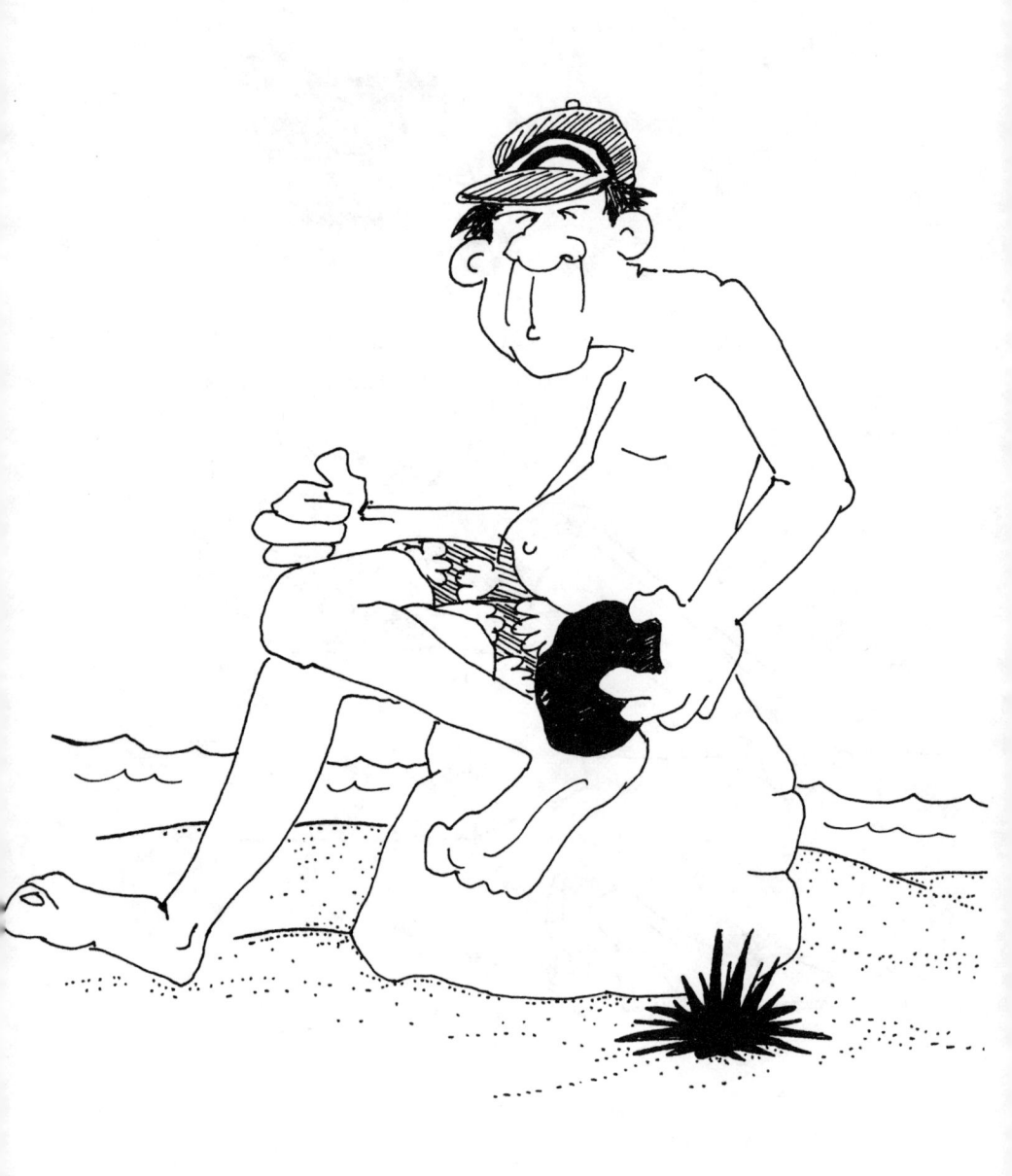

If you get a wana (sea urchin) spine in your foot, take a rock and crush the spine. Breaking up the spine makes it heal faster. (Only real men or real fools can do this).

Rub meat tenderizer into a Portuguese-man-of-war sting to prevent pain and swelling. If no tenderizer is available, pee on it. (Meat tenderizer contains papain, an enzyme which breaks down venom, and urine contains ammonia which relieves itching.)

If you get a wana spine in your foot, soak it in vinegar.

Place crushed laukāhi leaves on wana spine wounds to ease the pain.

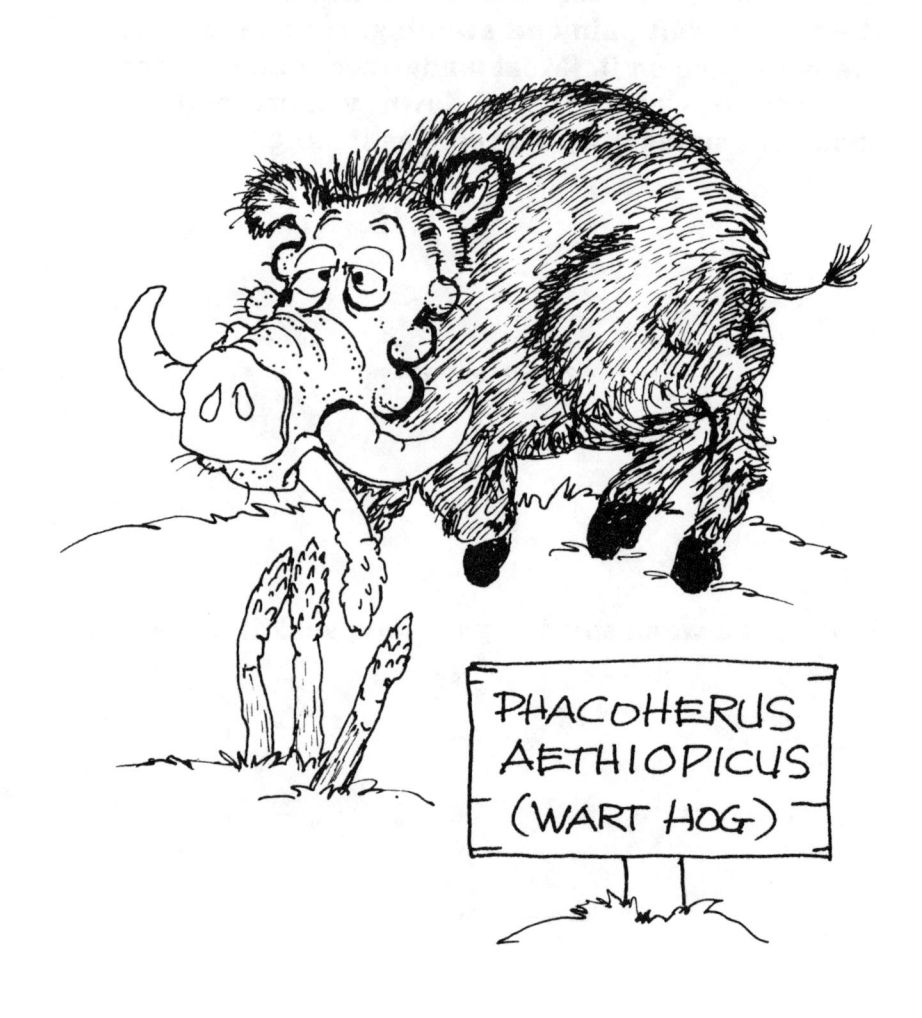

Eat lots of asparagus to remove warts.

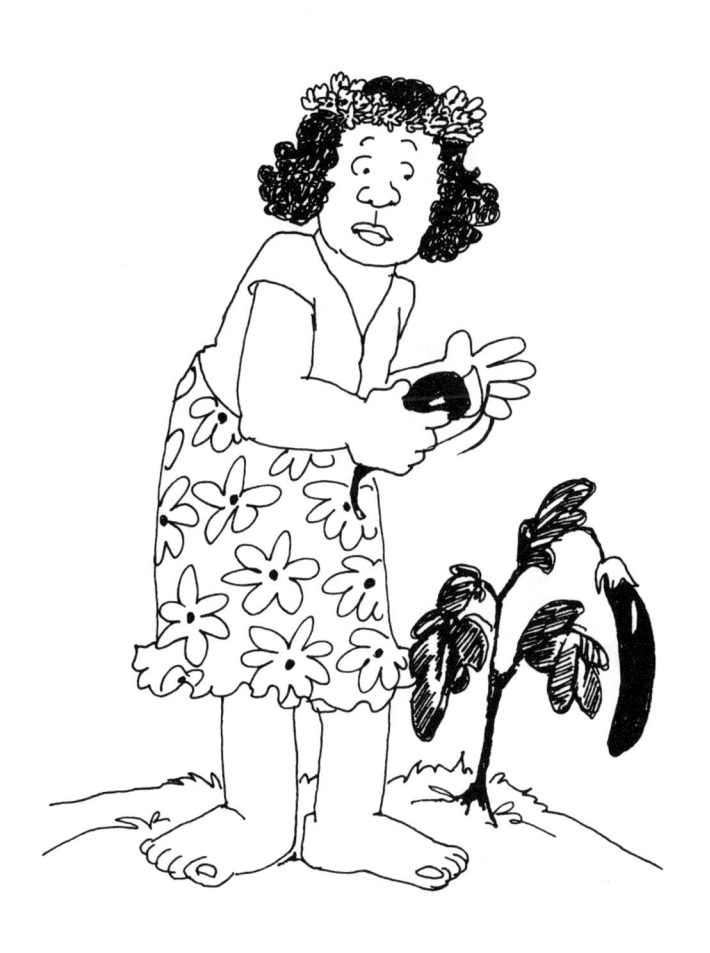

To remove a wart, rub a cut nasubi (Japanese eggplant) on it. Bury the nasubi in the ground and the wart will go away.

Apply mashed dandelion greens to warts to make them disappear.

To remove warts, apply the juice of mashed marigold flowers.

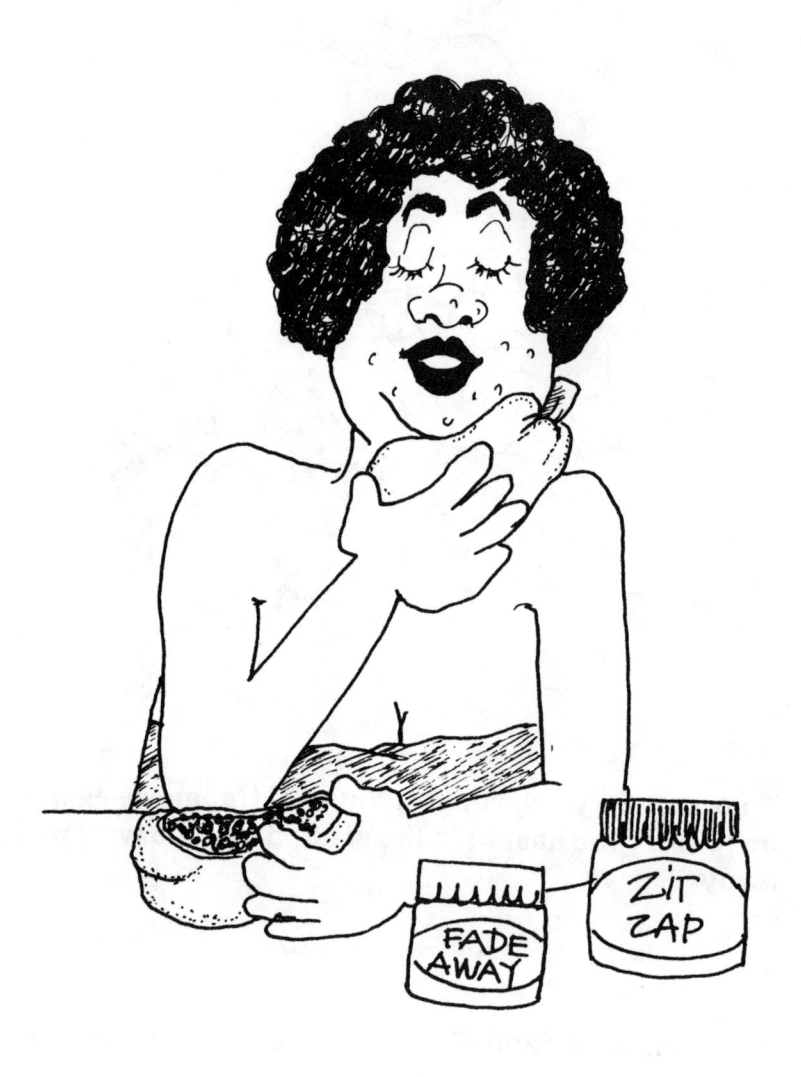

Rub the milky sap from the skin of green papaya on your skin to remove blemishes.

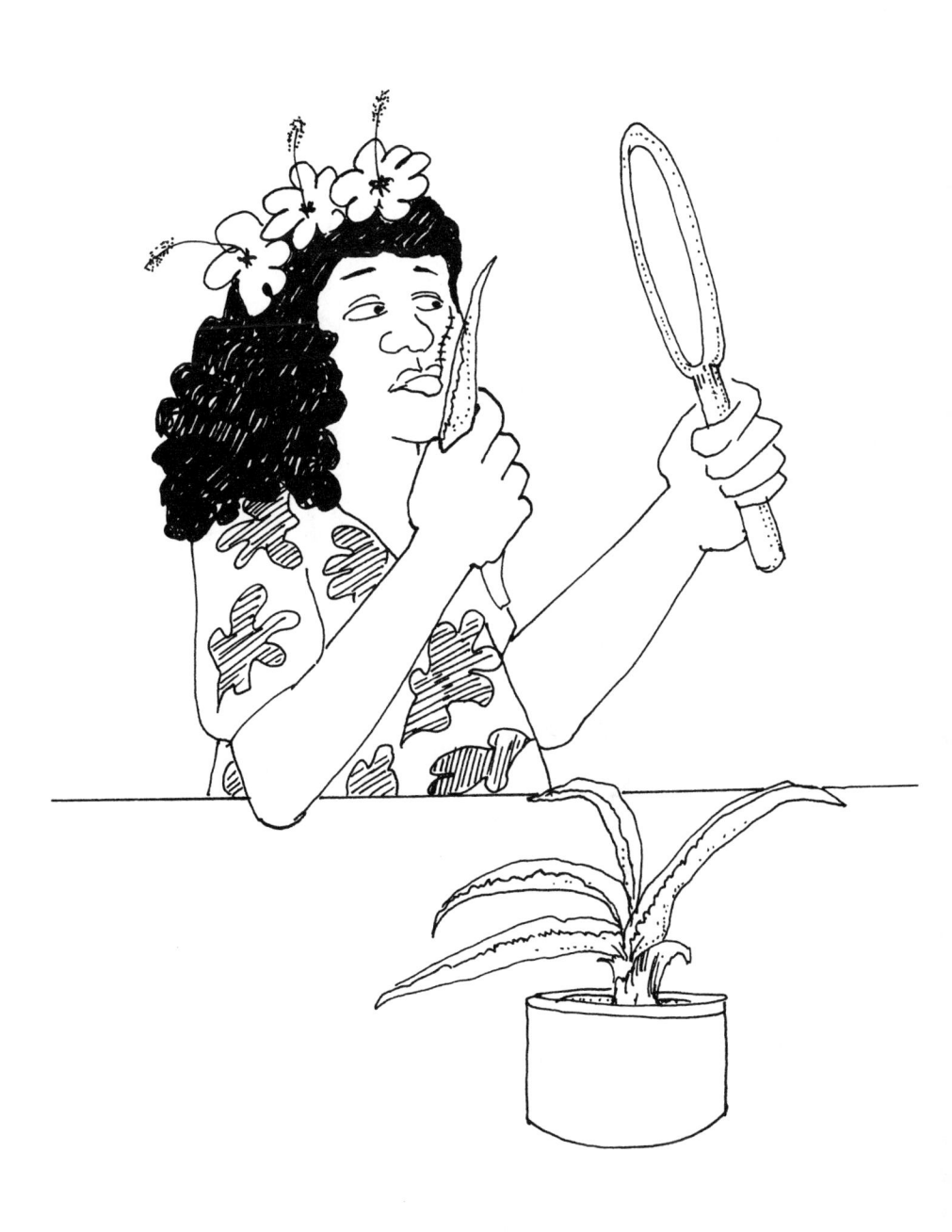

After surgery, rub the juice of aloe on a scar and you will have a beautiful scar rather than an ugly one.

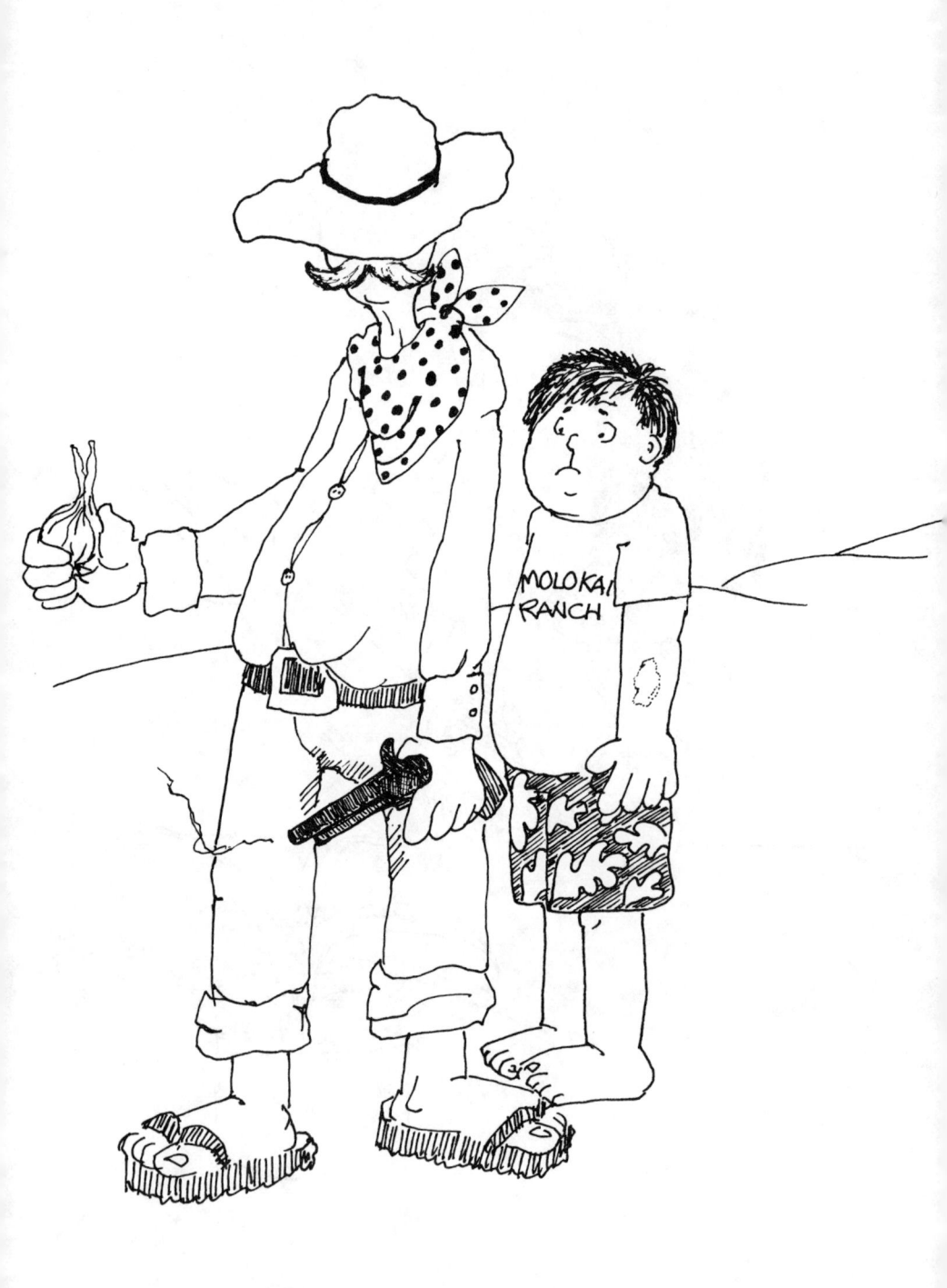

To get rid of ringworm, rub a mixture of gunpowder and garlic on it.

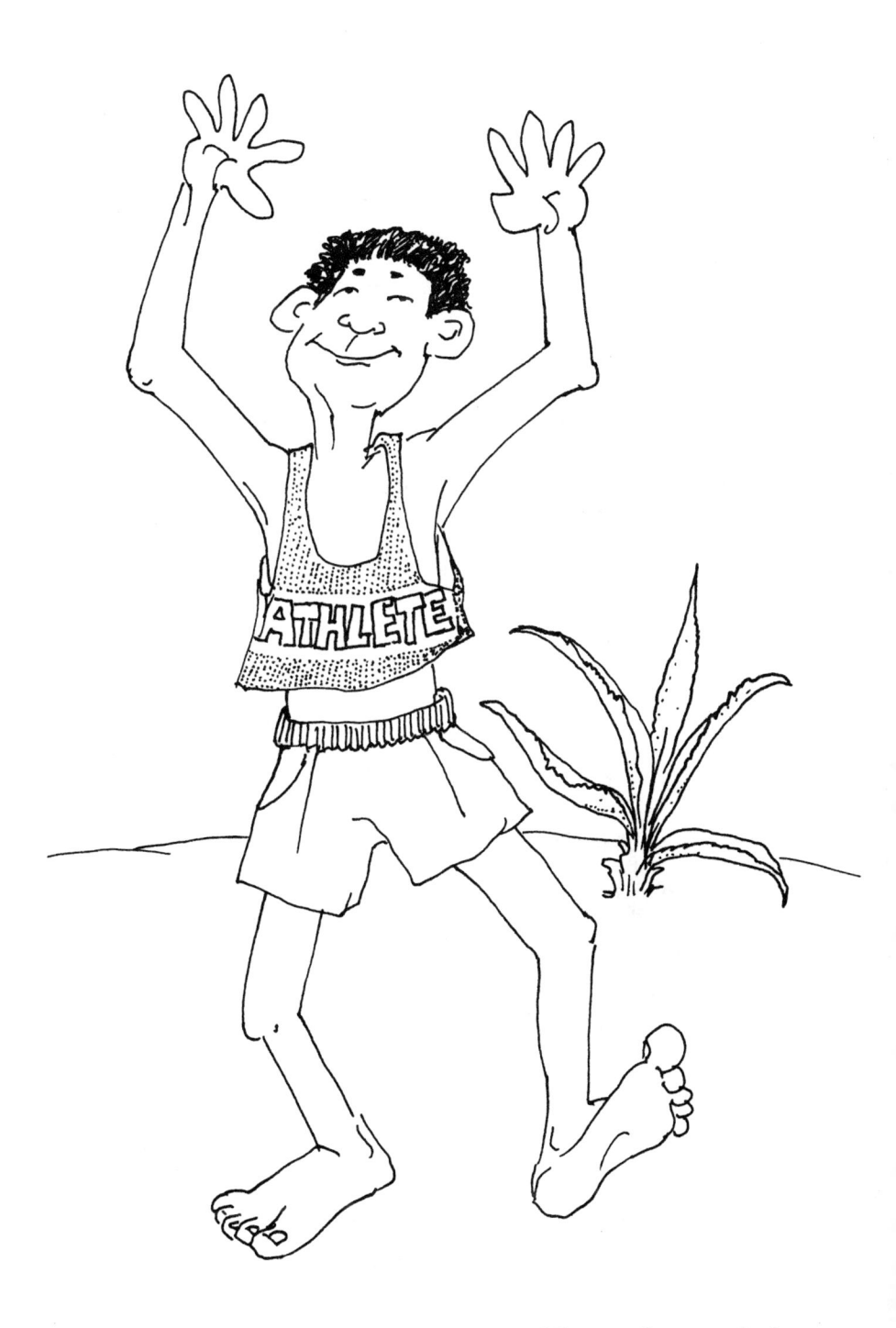

Use the juice from aloe to treat athlete's foot and ringworm.

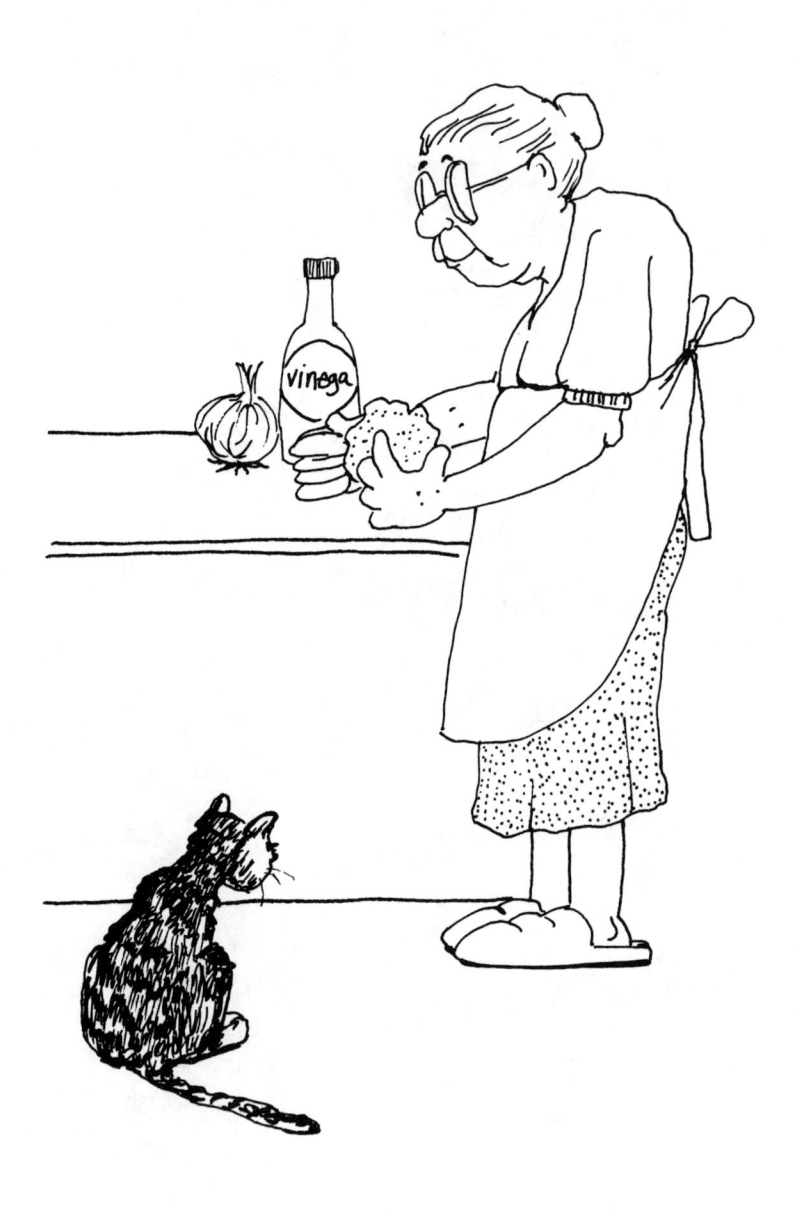

Onion juice and vinegar applied to the skin removes freckles and age spots.

Burns, Wounds, and Sores

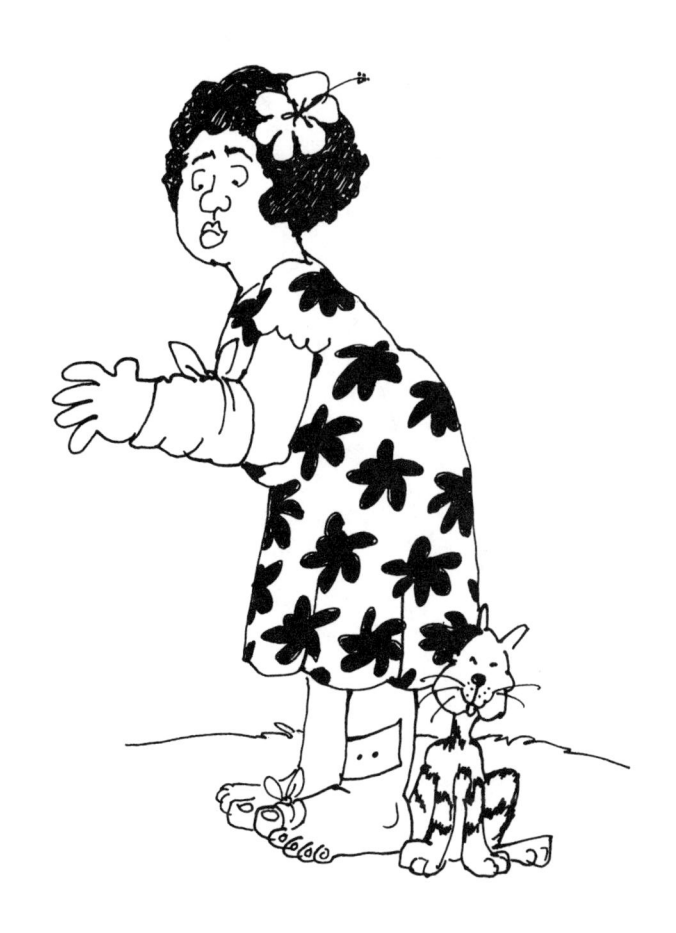

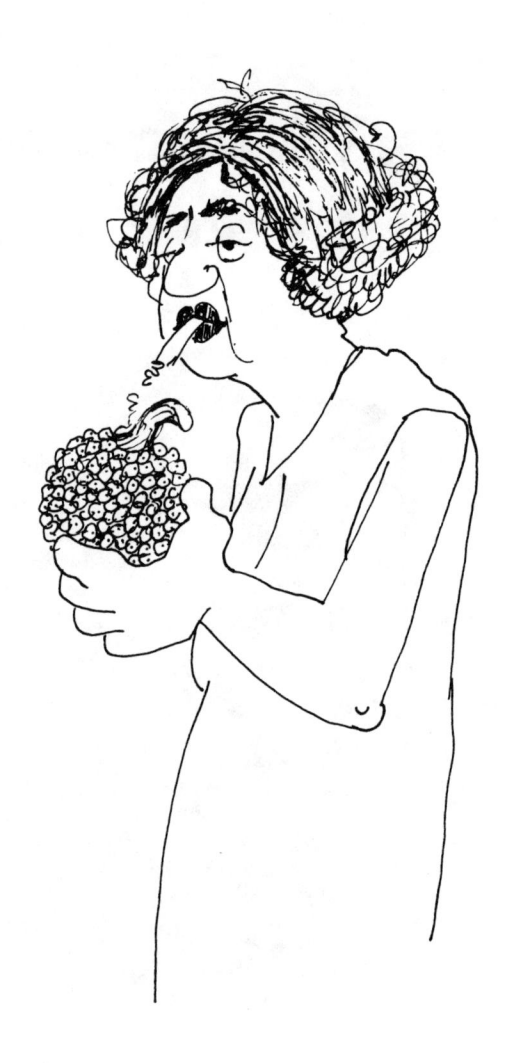

The sap from the stem of breadfruit mixed with tobacco ashes is effective for treating skin diseases and boils.

The milky sap from a papaya is good for cuts, open wounds, and sores.

Crushed māmaki berries help to heal sores and wounds.

Boil honeysuckle leaves in water to make a lotion to heal sores and wounds.

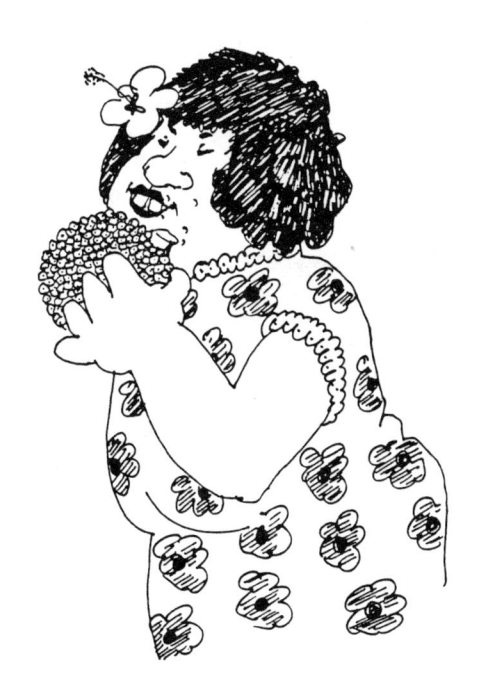

Use the sap from breadfruit for healing cuts, cracked or chapped skin, and scratches. Sores around the mouth are also relieved by this sap.

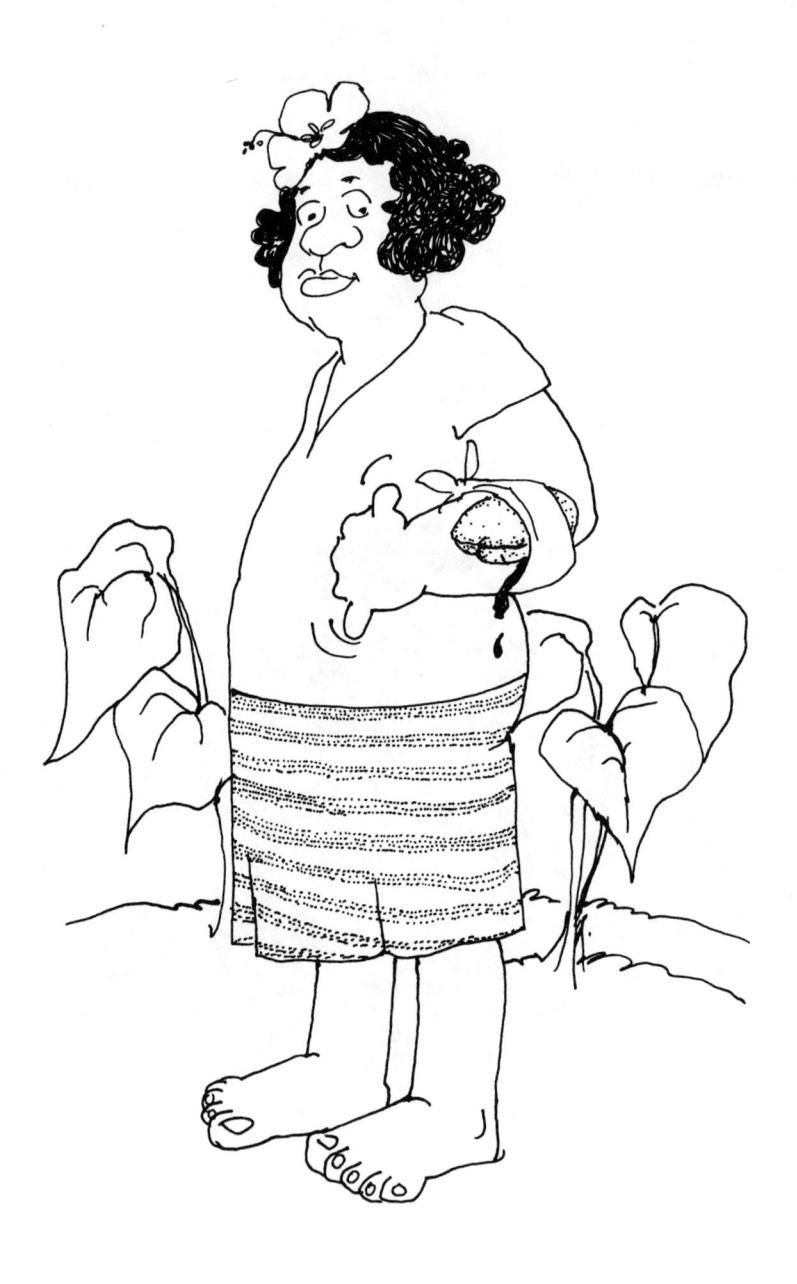

Hawaiian band-aid: Tie a raw taro slice on a wound. It stops the bleeding.

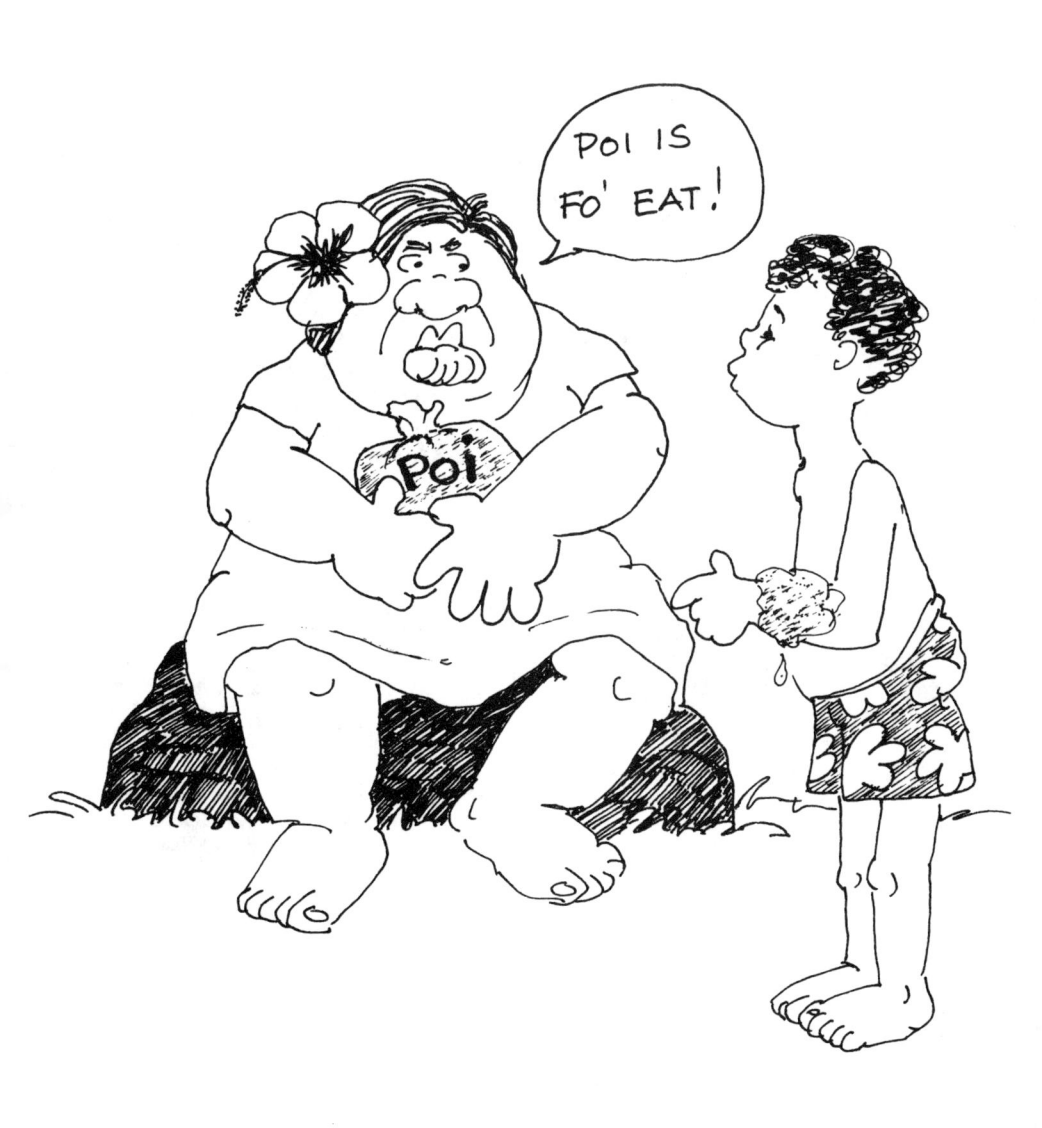

Unmixed or undiluted poi can be used as a poultice on infected sores.

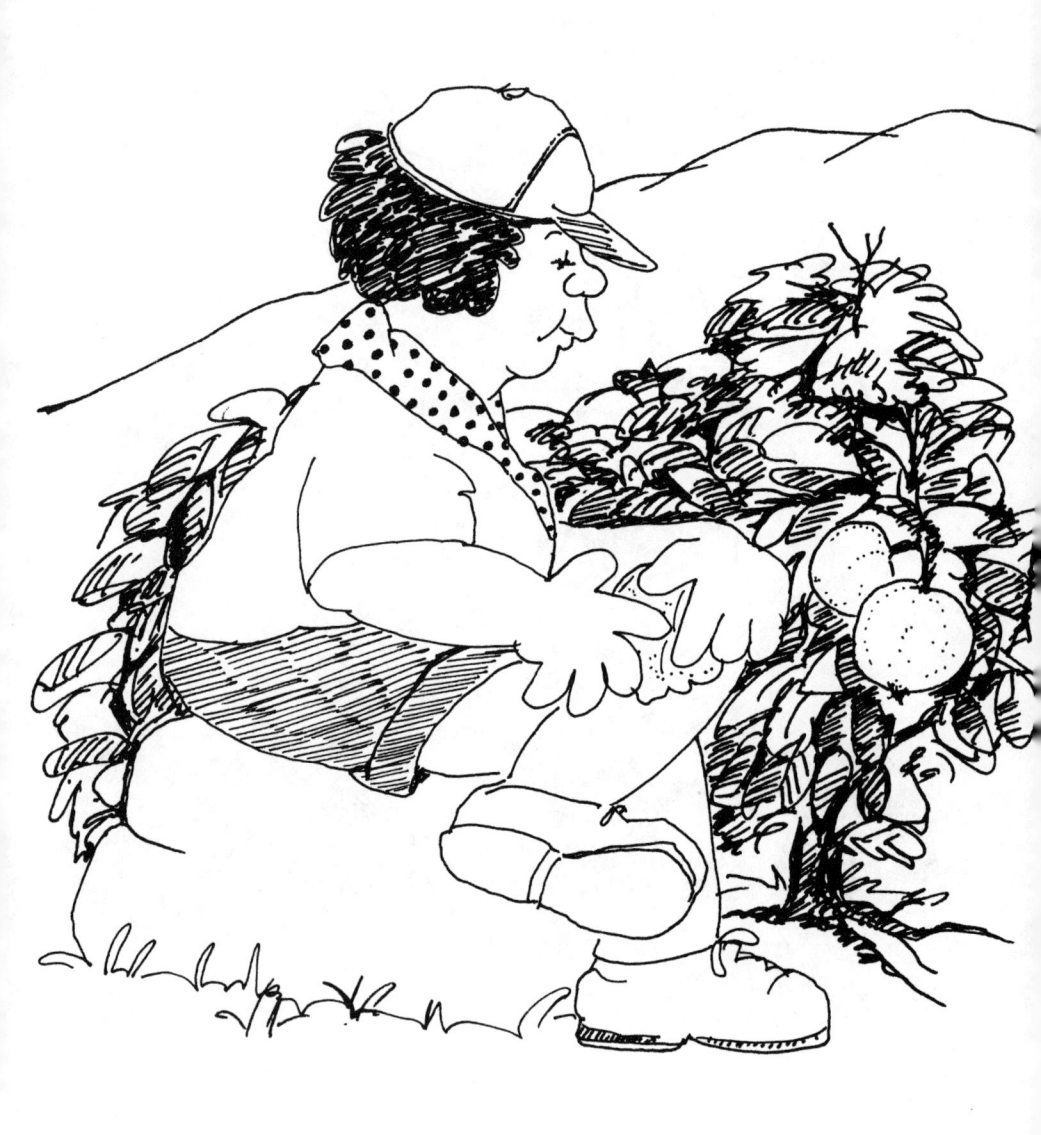

If you get a cut while hiking, chew some guava leaves until they are finely crushed. Place the leaves on the wound and bind them in place with a bandage made out of the fibrous part of the guava fruit.

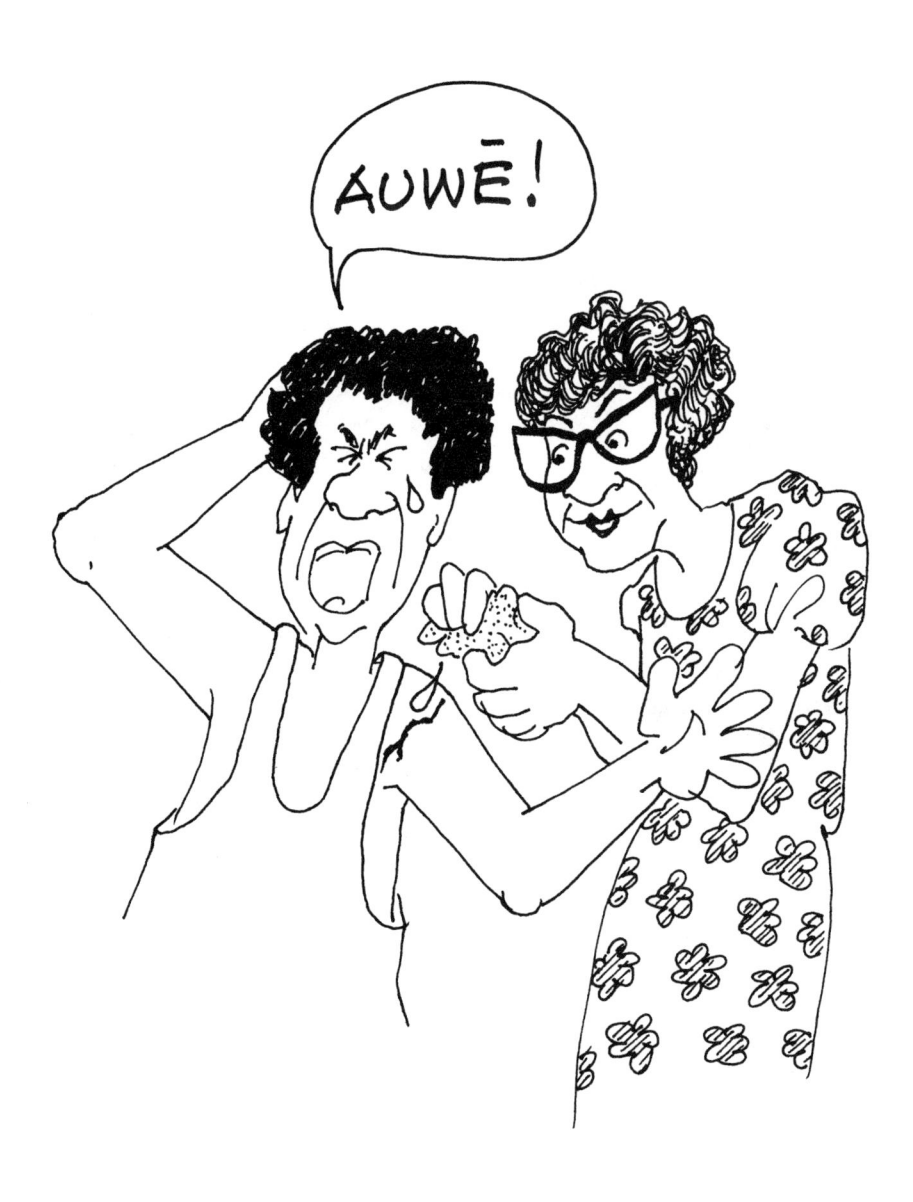

For deep cuts, take 2 pieces of bark from a mountain apple tree and mix them with a handful of Hawaiian salt. Wrap in a thin cloth and squeeze the juice onto the wound.

Honohono grass (wandering Jew) applied to a wound will stop bleeding.

Crush leaves of pōpolo, mix with Hawaiian salt, and apply it to cuts.

Pound unripe noni fruit with Hawaiian salt and put it on deep cuts and compound fractures.

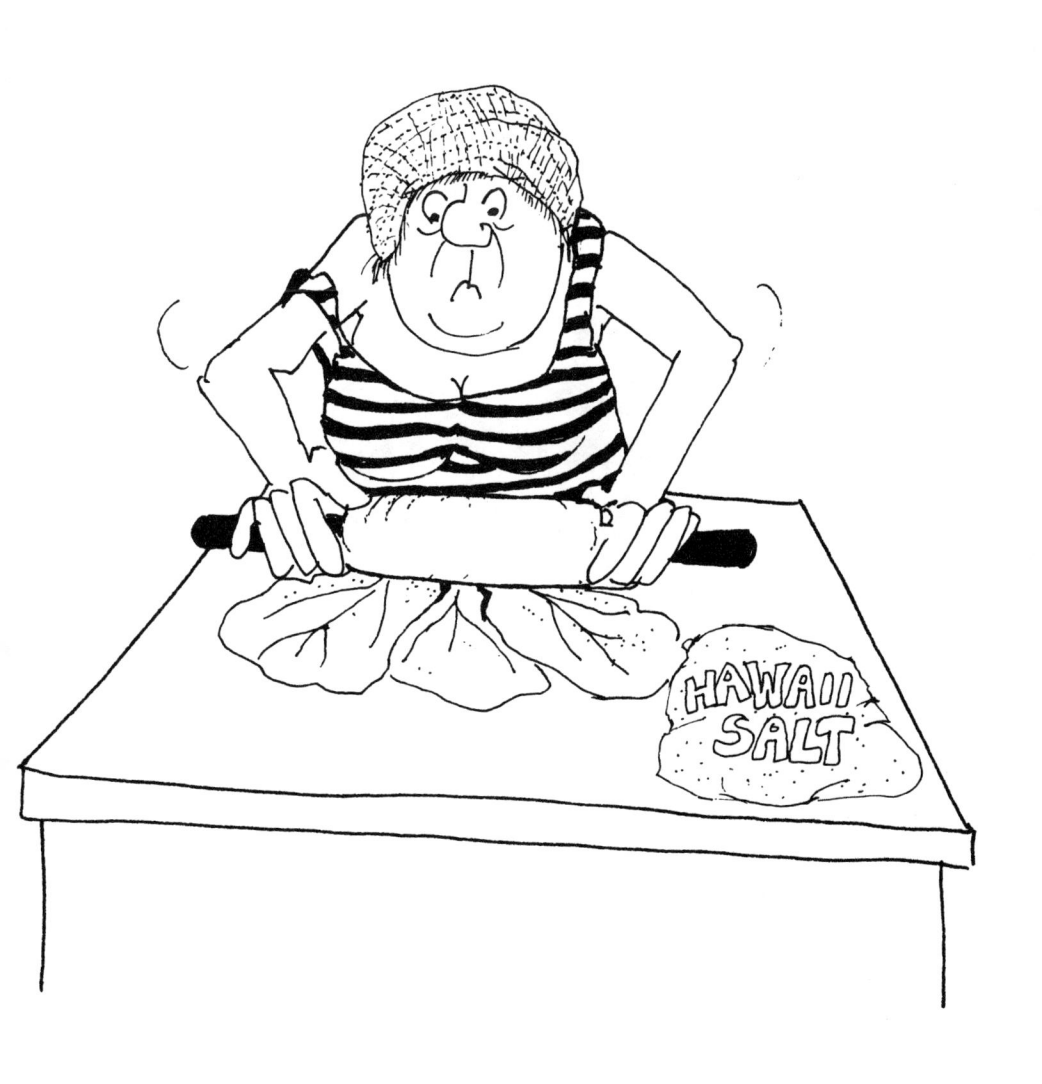

To hasten healing of a boil, take laukāhi leaves, sprinkle them with Hawaiian salt and mash the salt into the leaves with a rolling pin. Bind the leaves onto the boil.

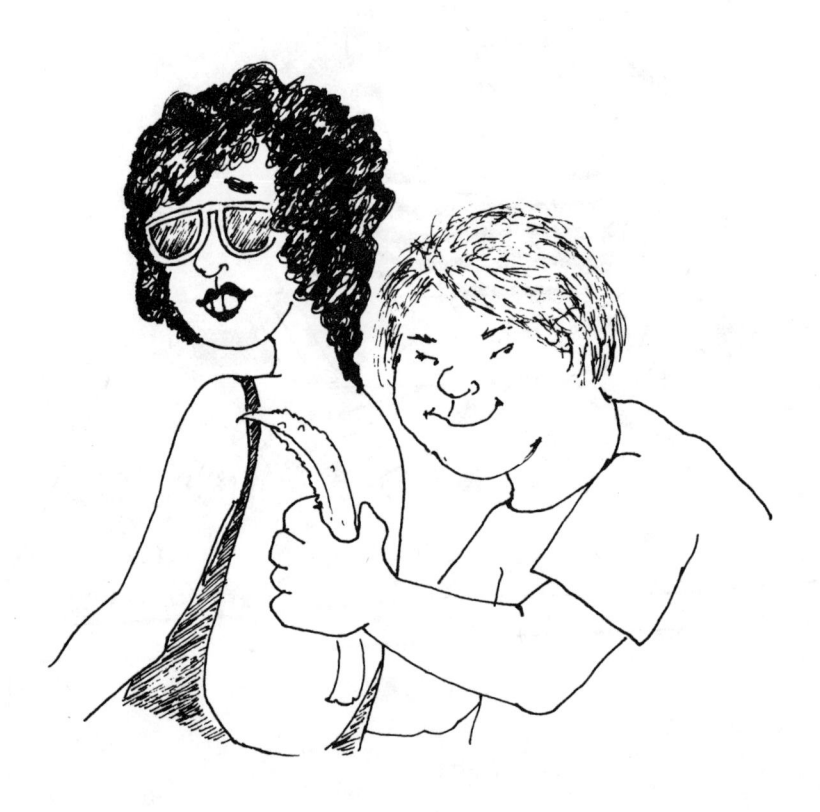

The juice of aloe heals cuts, burns, and scrapes. If rubbed on minor burns and sunburn immediately, your skin will not blister.

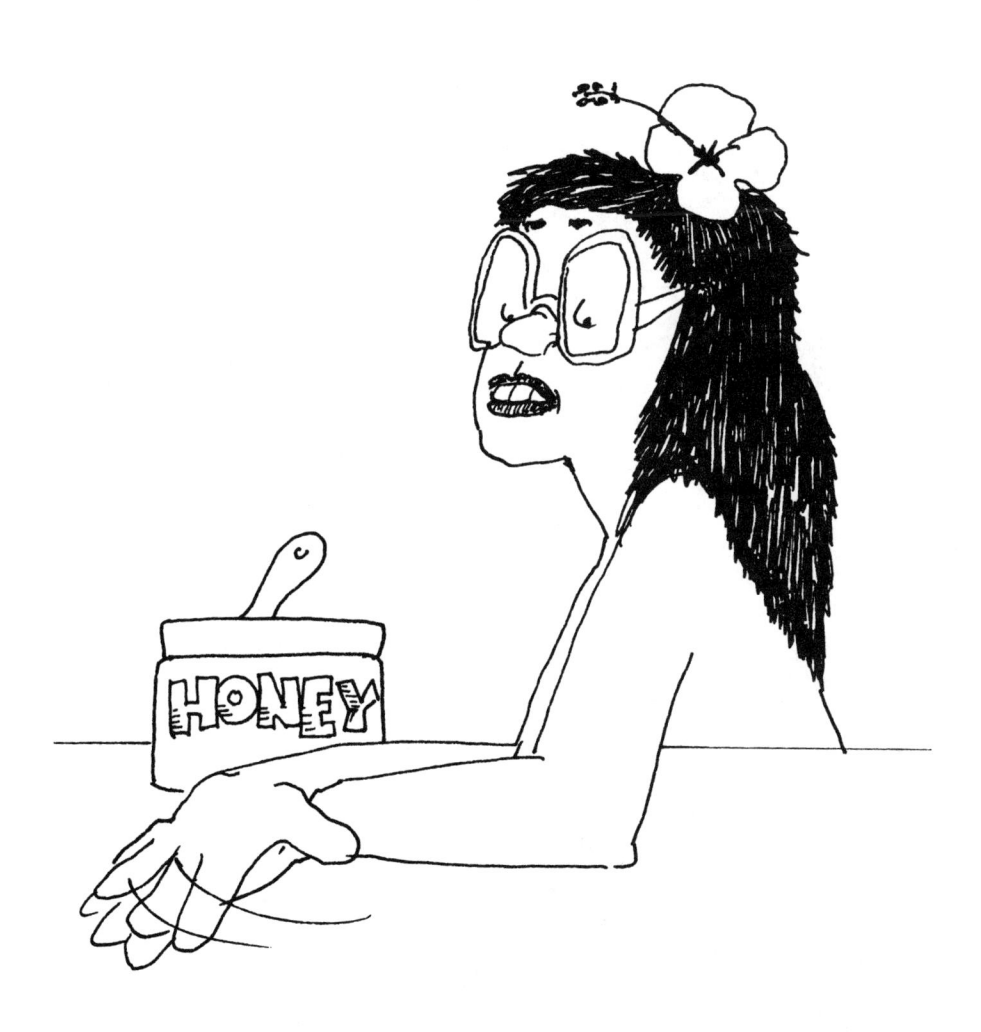

Honey is an effective treatment for minor burns.

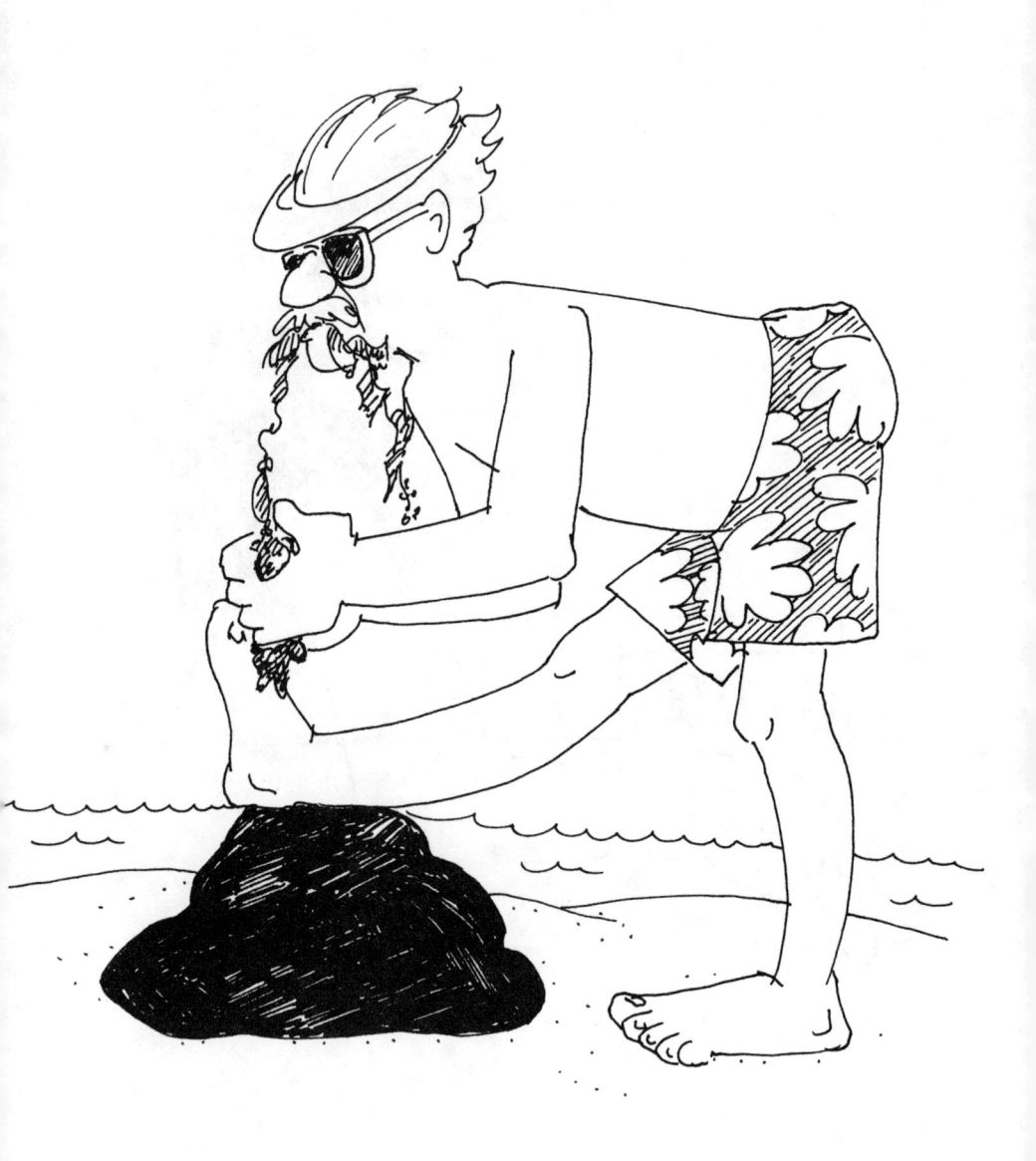

If you get a coral cut, chop or chew limu kala (common yellow-brown seaweed) and apply it to the wound.

Coughs, Colds, and Fever

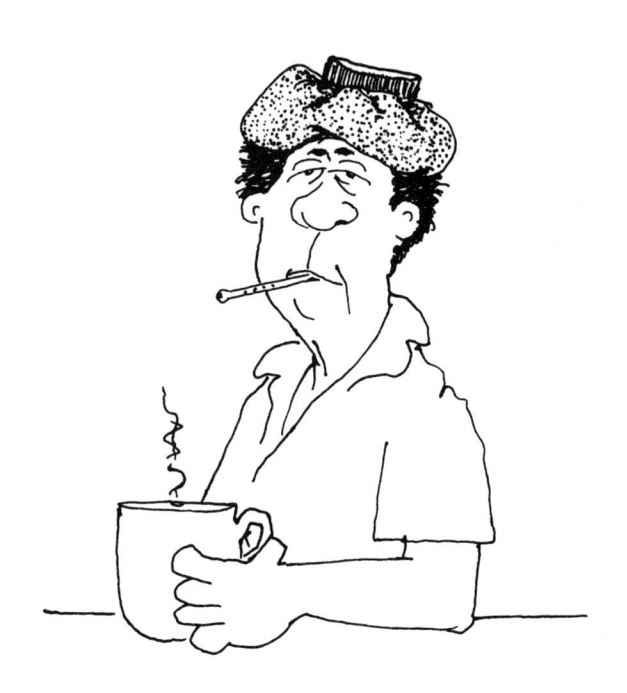

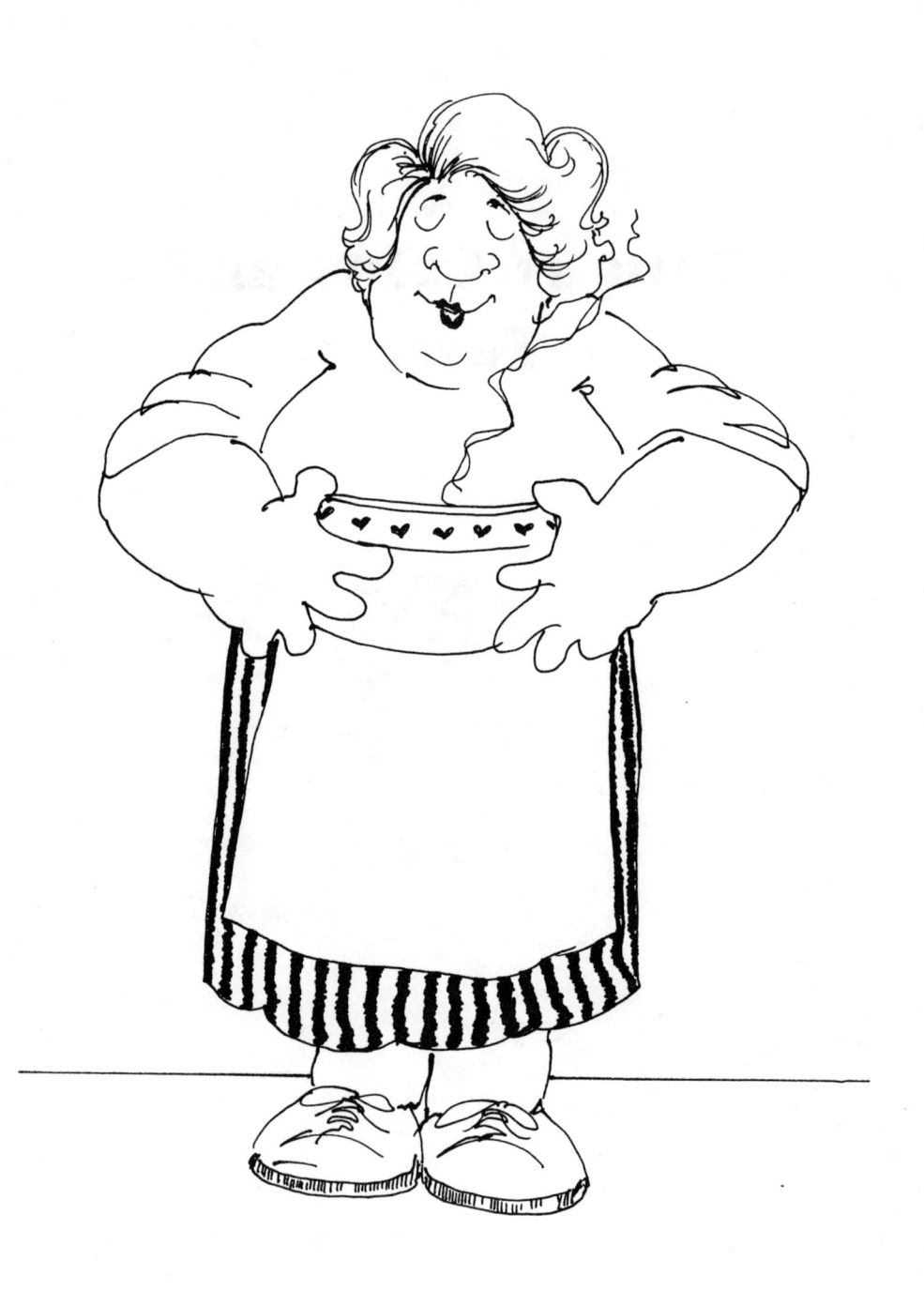

When you have a cold, eat chicken soup. It helps to get rid of cold organisms naturally.

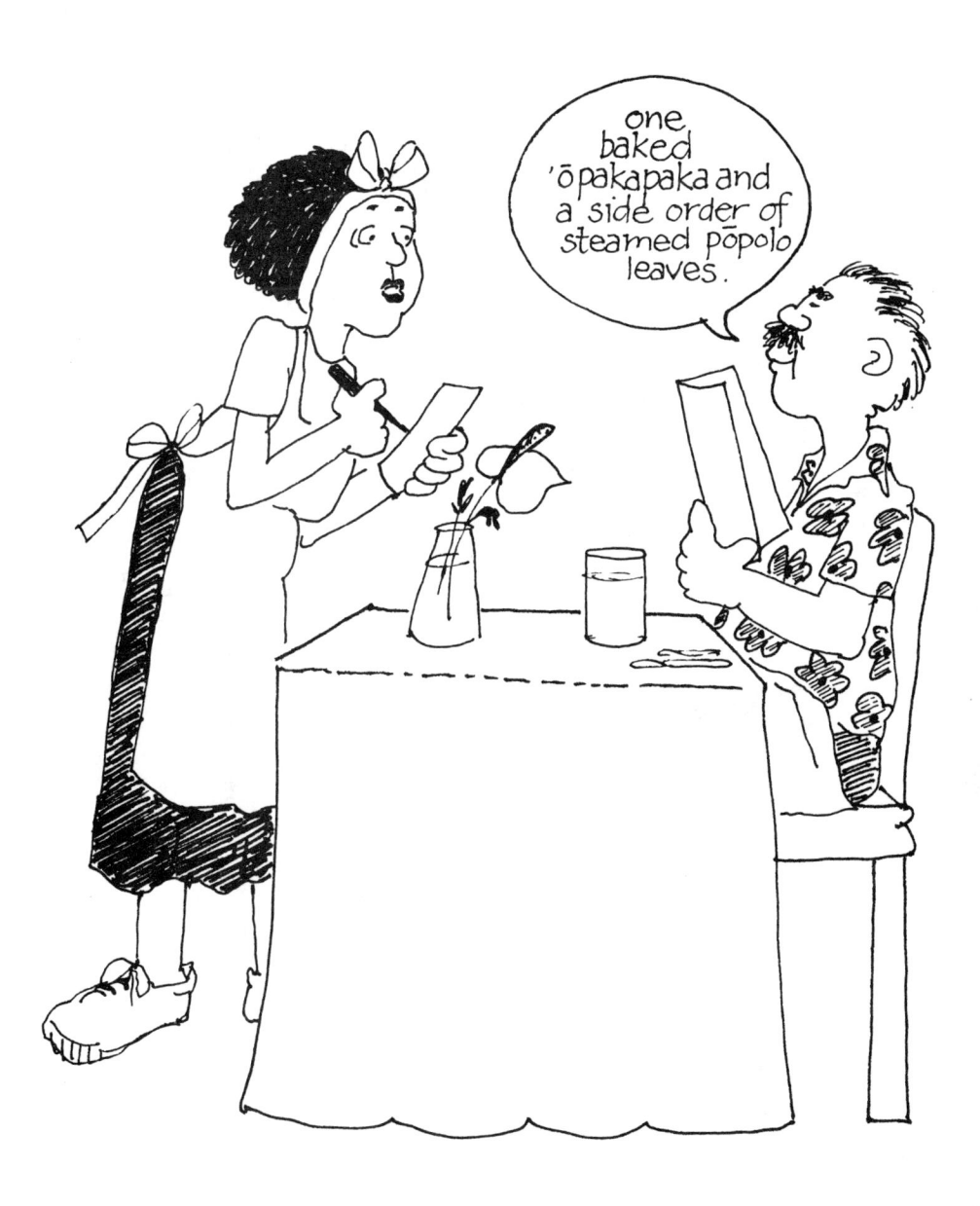

To relieve a cold, steam some pōpolo leaves wrapped in a ti leaf. Discard the ti leaf, divide the popolo leaves in 5 equal parts and eat them with your dinner for 5 consecutive days.

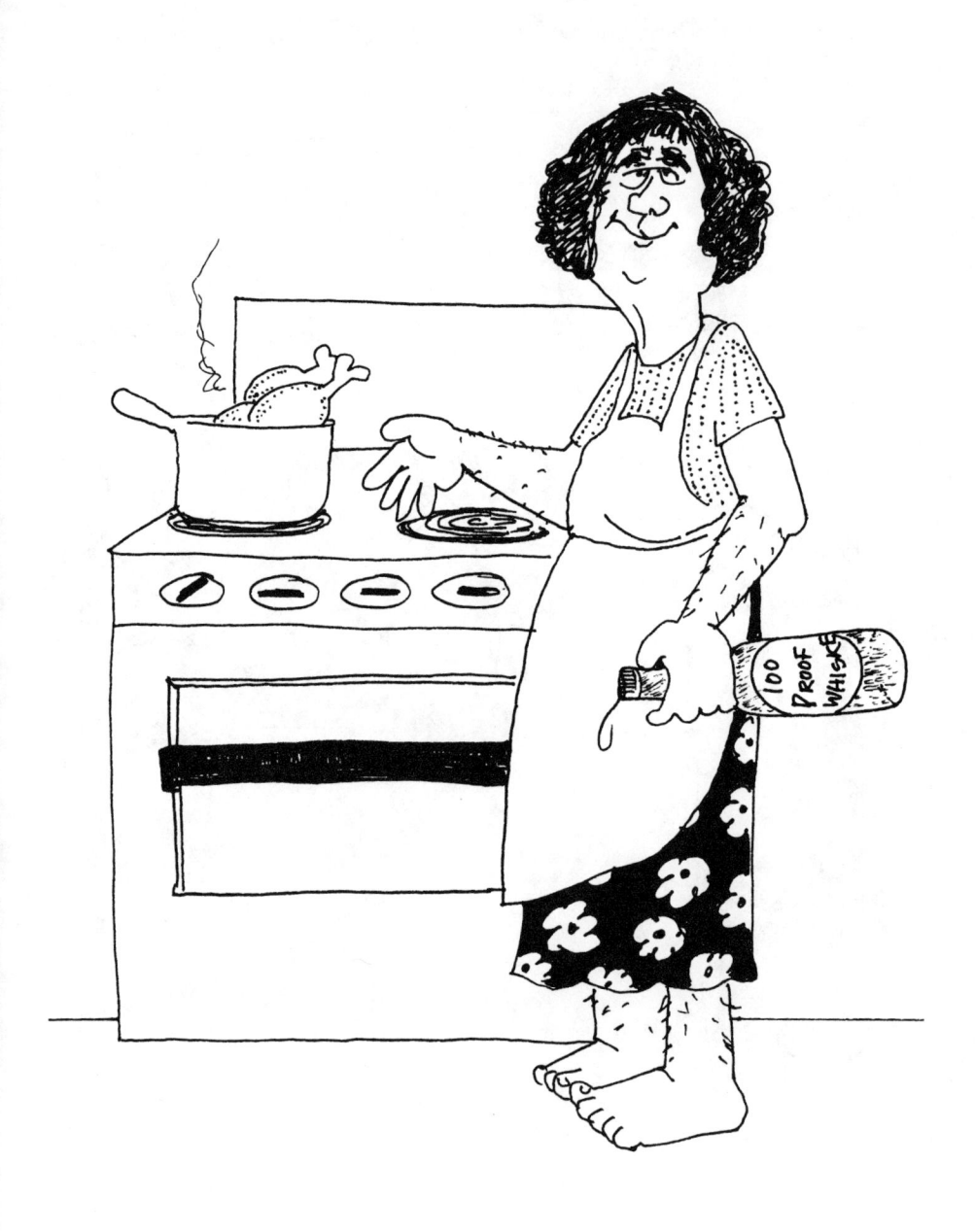

Okinawan chicken soup will cure a cold. Take 1 chicken, pour a quart of whiskey over it, and simmer. Drink the broth, but don't eat the chicken.

A cup of hot tea with an ume (Japanese pickled plum) in it will cure a cold.

If you feel a cold coming on, chew a piece of raw onion, holding it at the back of the mouth for a few minutes.

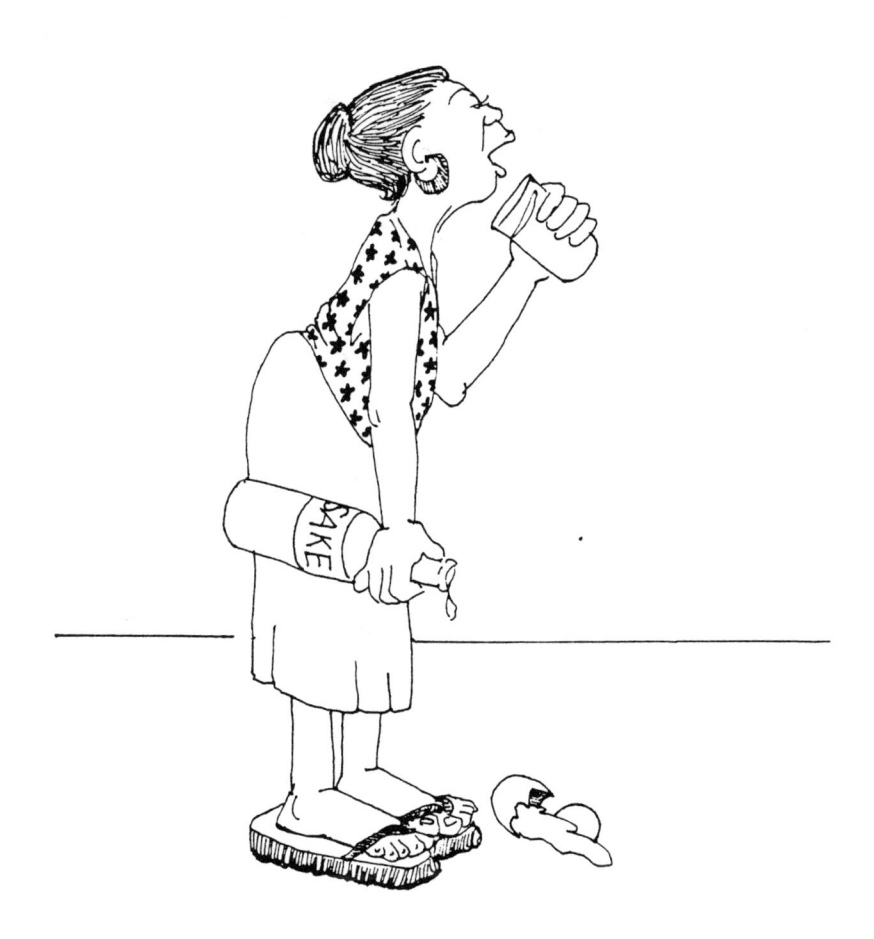

Drink a pint of hot sake with 1 egg yolk beaten in it to cure a cold.

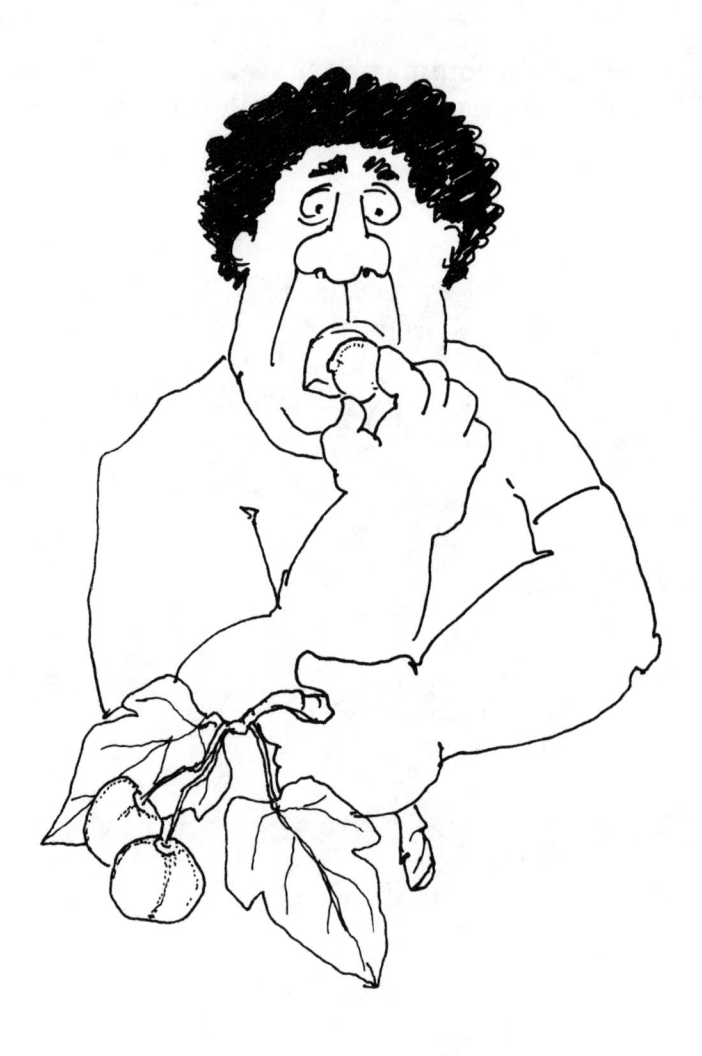

To relieve the pain of cold sores, rub the meat of a kukui nut on them.

Fresh pineapple helps to soothe a sore throat.

Rub vinegar on cold sores to relieve pain and discomfort.

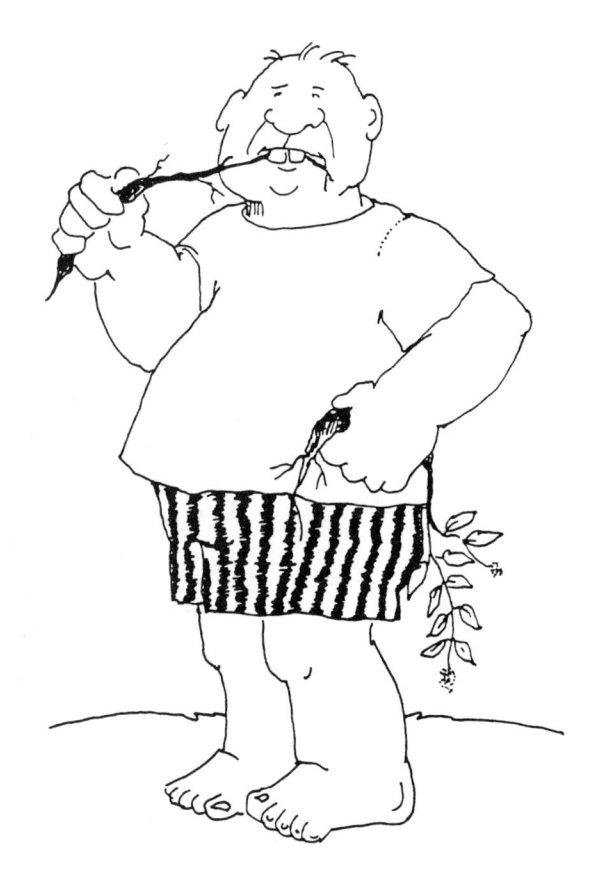

Chew roots of 'uhaloa (or make tea out of it) to soothe a sore throat.

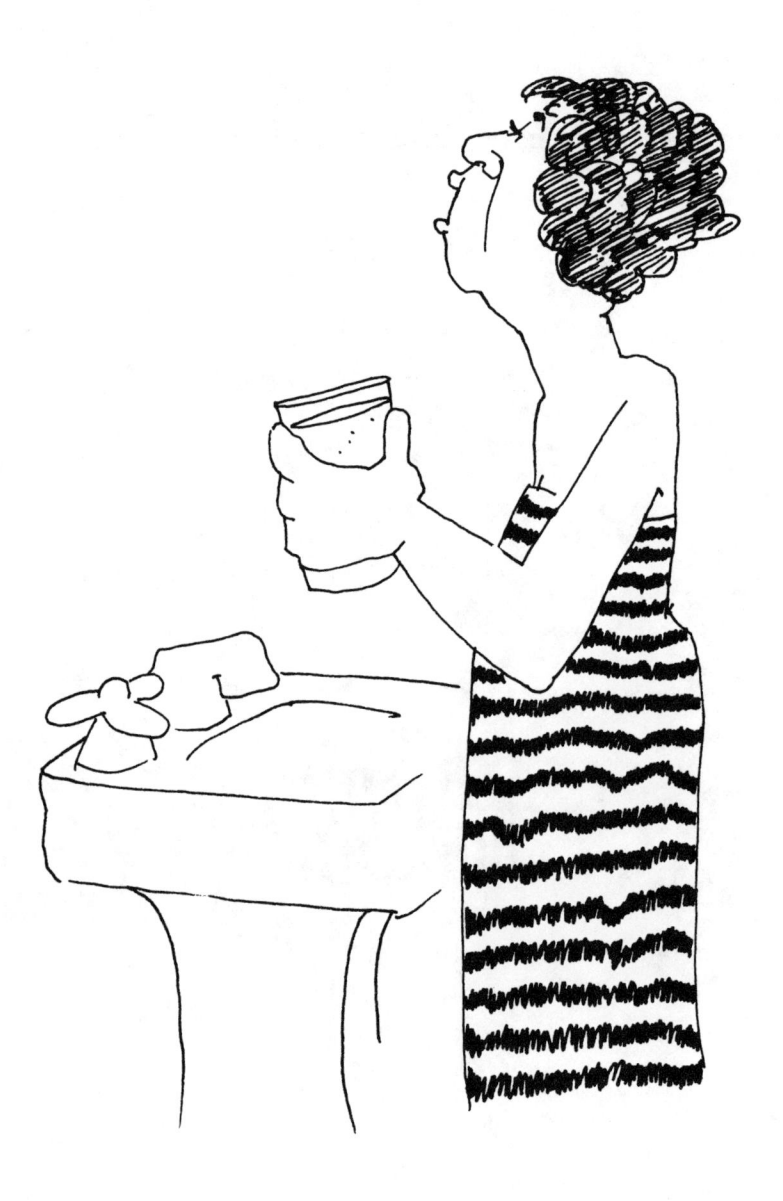

Gargle with sea water to soothe a sore throat.

If you have a sore throat, boil some bark of a mango tree and gargle with the liquid.

Gargling with a tea made out of boiling Chinese ginger in water soothes a sore throat.

Peel and dry pomelo (jabon) skin and keep it on hand. Boil it in water and gargle with the liquid when you have a sore throat.

For a sore throat or tonsillitis, cut a pomegranate in half, boil it in water, cool, and gargle with this juice.

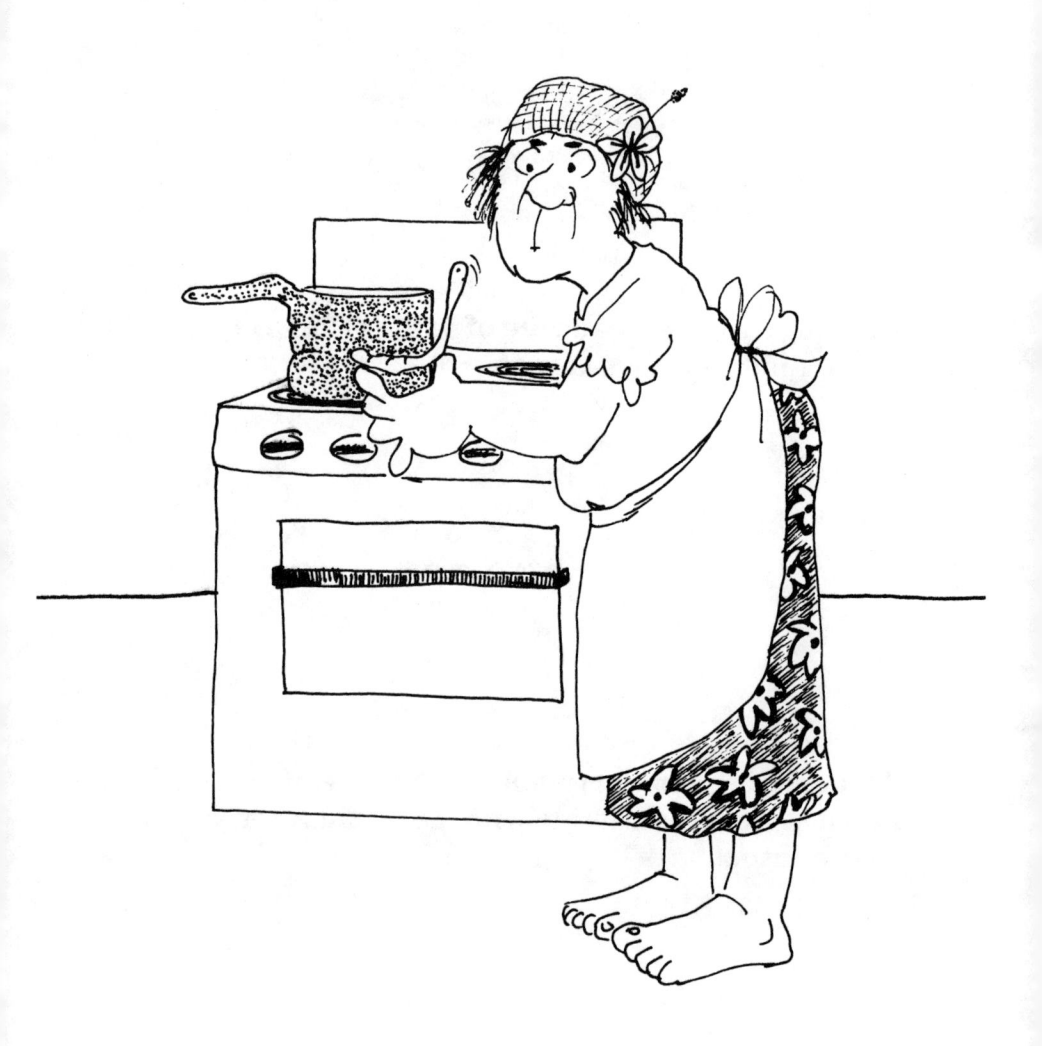

To get rid of a lingering fever, take 3 earthworms (turn the inside out with a chopstick to remove the dirt), and simmer them in water with a handful of hay. Drink a small cup of this "tea" several times a day.

Honeysuckle blossoms can be used like aspirin. Boil the flowers in water and drink the juice.

To reduce a high fever, take a handful of nanten (nandina), wash it with salt, and place in some water. When the water turns a pale green, give a tablespoon to the sick person. Repeat every hour if necessary.

1 tablespoon of blood from a live carp will reduce fever.

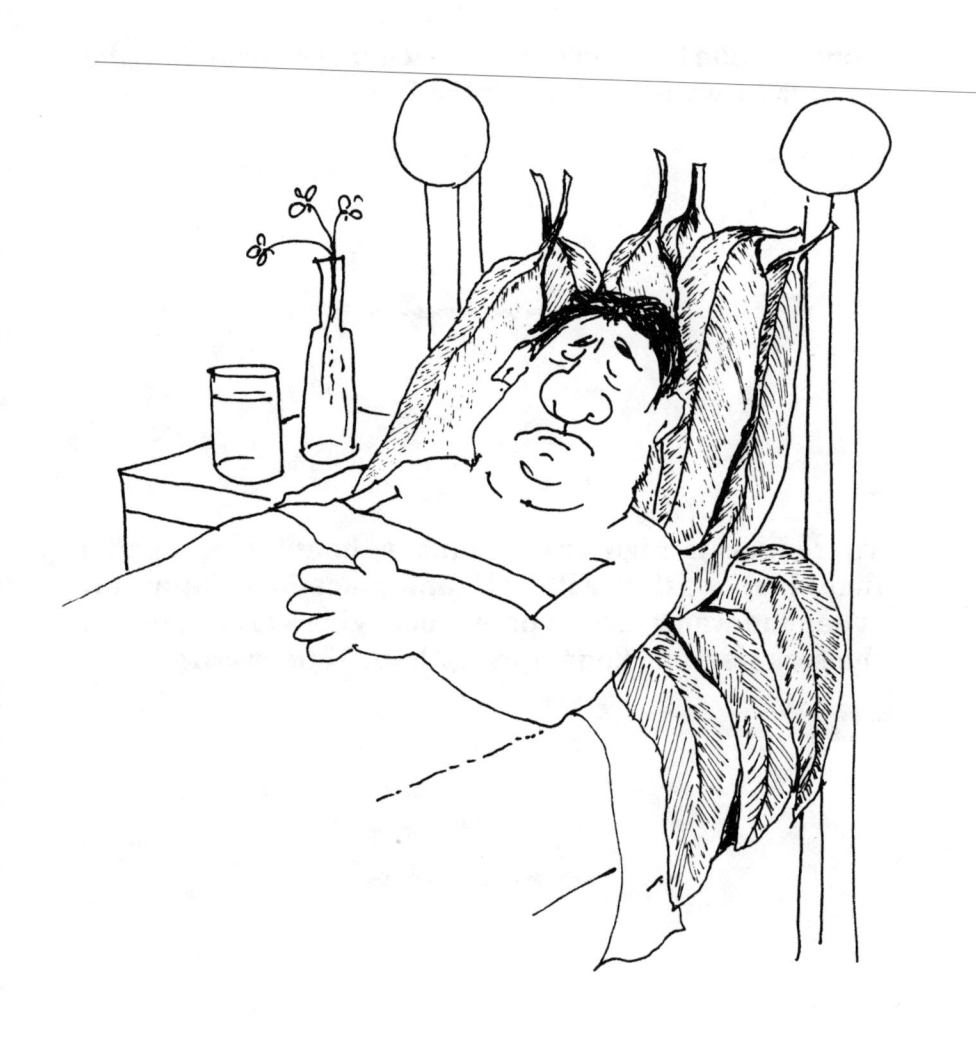

If a person has a high fever, line his bed with ti leaves.
The leaves will draw the fever out of him.

A tonic made out of 'awa soaked in water and mixed with mountain apple leaves and buds, the outside of a green kukui nut, and a bit of sugar cane relieves chills and fever.

Boil pōpolo berries and drink the liquid to keep fever down.

Boil leaves and stems of Chinese taro in water for 1 hour or more. Drink this juice for a high fever.

To calm a feverish child, chew leaf buds of 'awa with some ilima flowers and give it to the child twice a day.

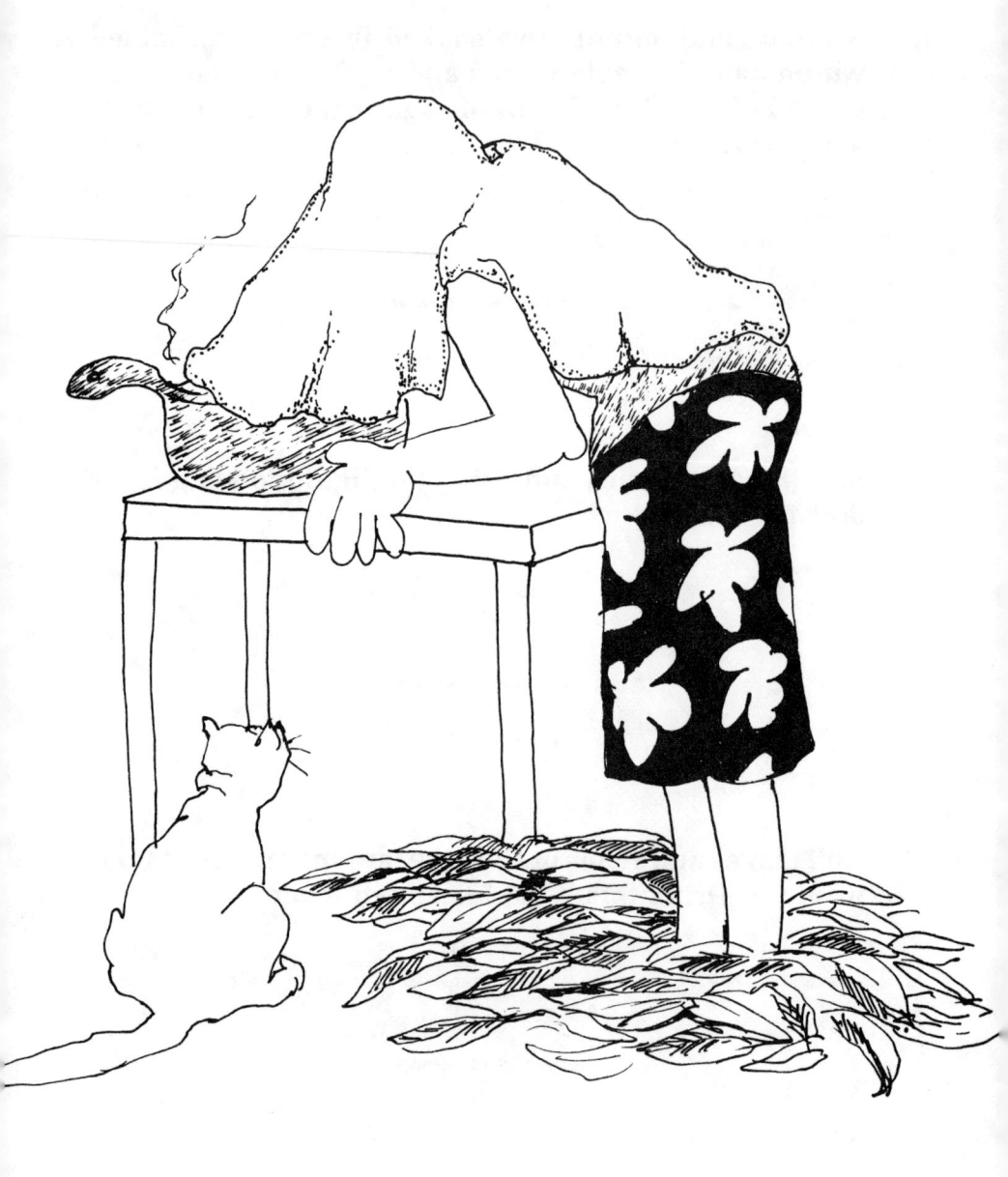

If your cheeks ache from sinus pressure, or if you have nasal congestion or a cough, drink an ounce of whiskey or other strong liquor. Collect about 40 eucalyptus leaves and boil them in a gallon of water. Put a cloth over your head and inhale the vapors. Repeat the treatment twice a day.

Boil a dozen lady slipper blossoms in water. Strain and drink the liquid to relieve coughs.

Boil dandelion greens in water until the liquid is reduced to one-half the original volume. This drink is good for colds, bronchitis, pneumonia, or any respirator ailment.

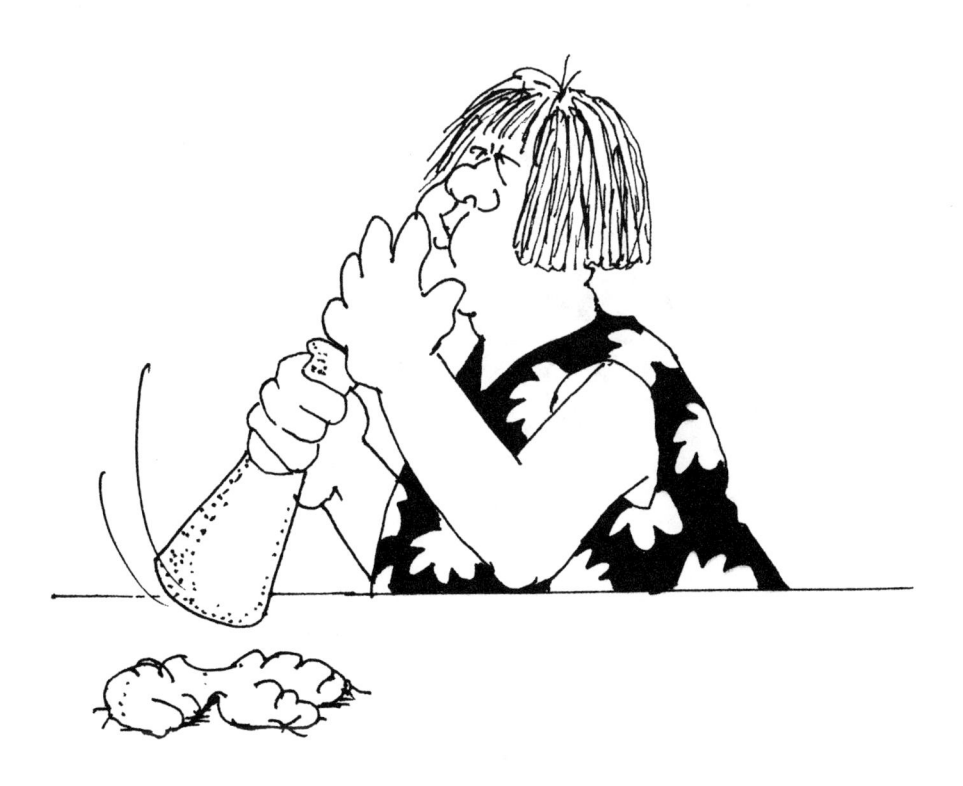

For a persistent cough, pound Chinese ginger root and mix its juice with honey. Take a spoonful as needed.

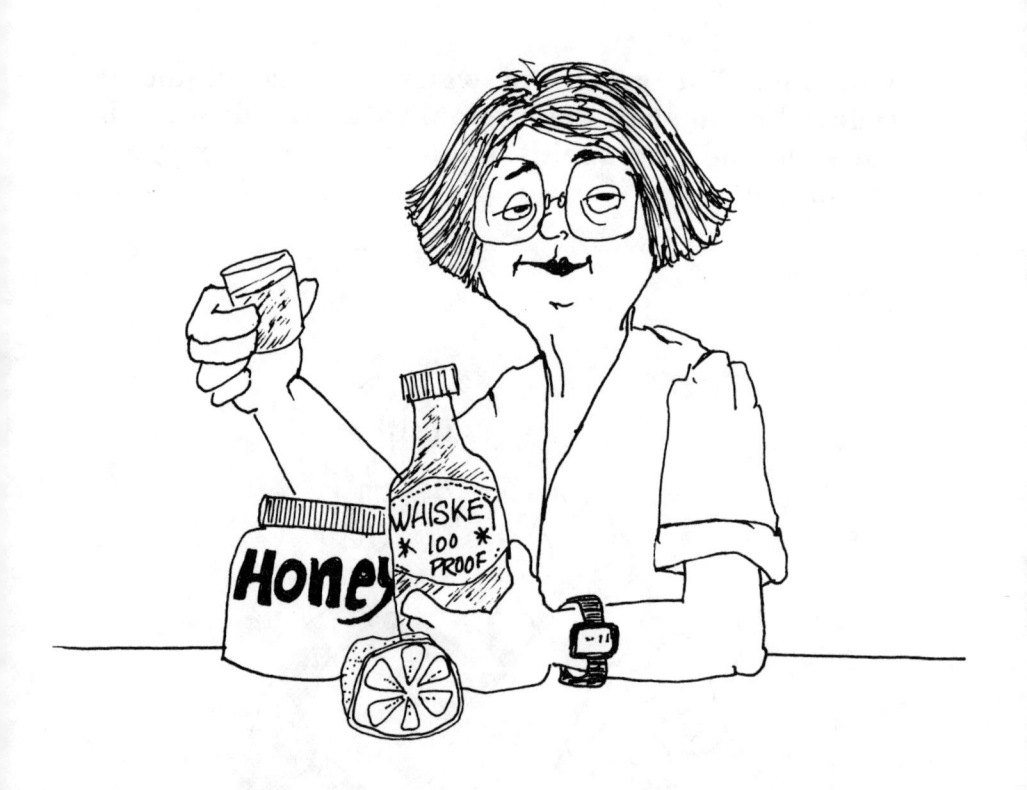

For cough medicine, take the juice of a lemon or an orange, mix it with a bit of honey and a jigger of whiskey.

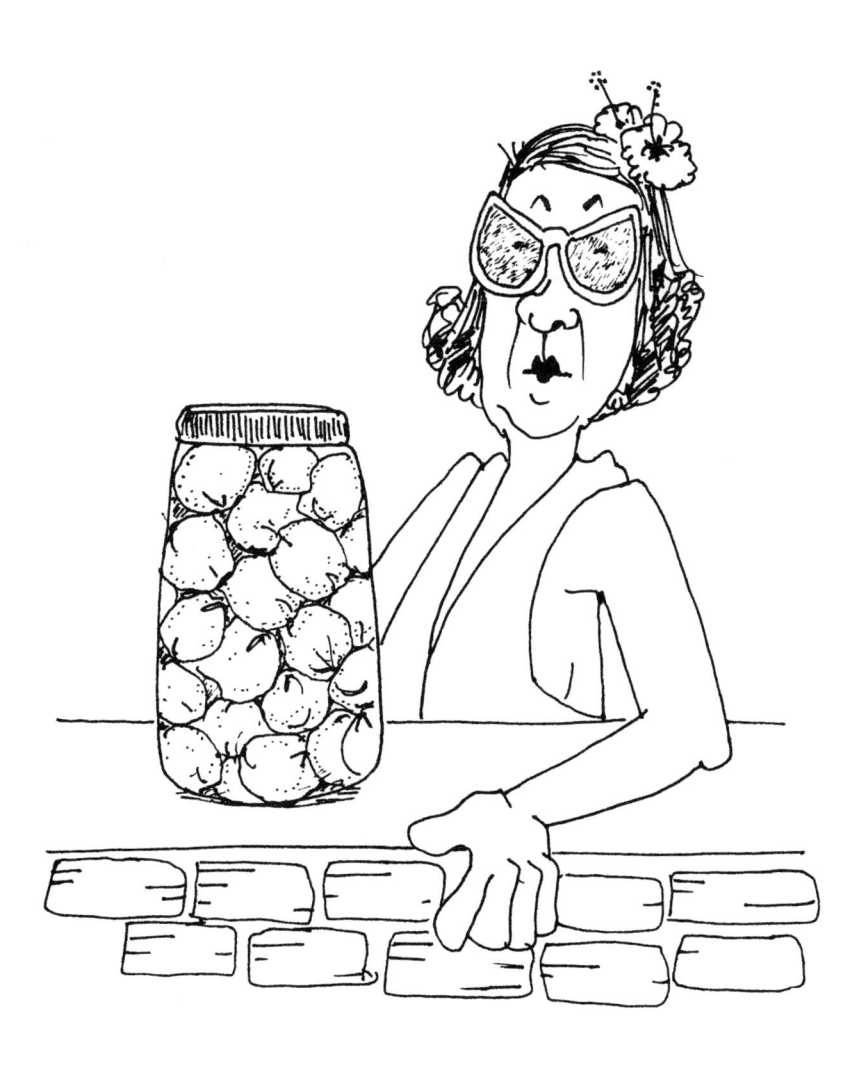

Put limes in a jar, sprinkle them with Hawaiian salt, cover and leave in the sun for several days. These preserved limes are good for coughs or sore throats. They may be eaten or put in a cup of hot tea.

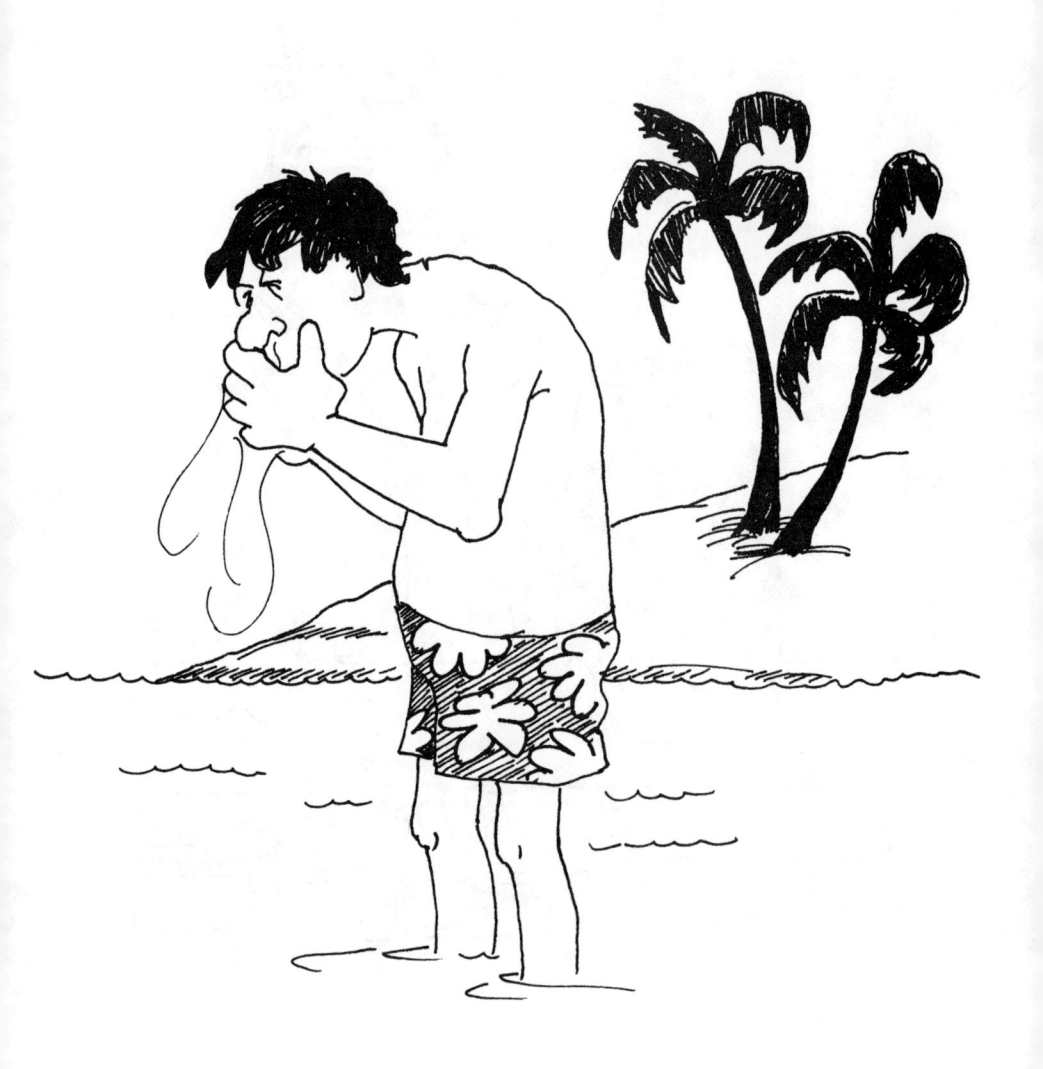

To clear sinus trouble, take some sea water in your cupped hands and sniff it up your nose 5 times a day until the problem is gone.

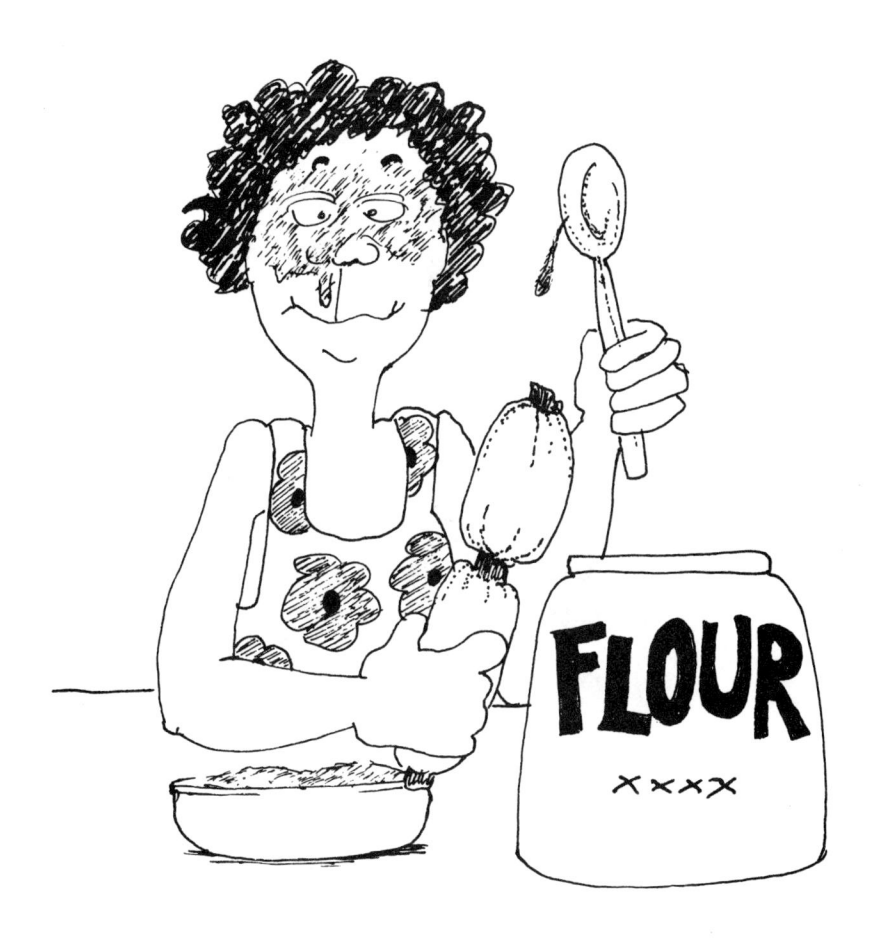

Make a paste out of grated fresh hasu (lotus root) and flour. Apply the mixture to the lower forehead and around the eyes to relieve sinus problems.

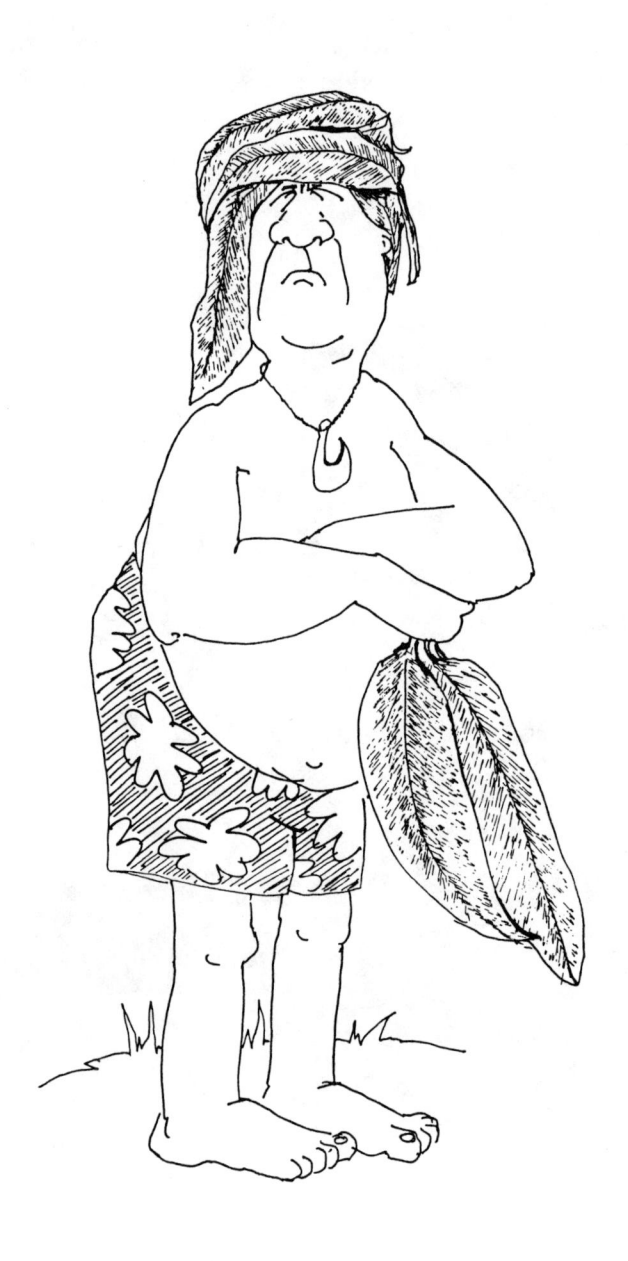

To get rid of a headache due to a cold, wrap ti leaves or 'awa leaves around your head.

Head Stuff

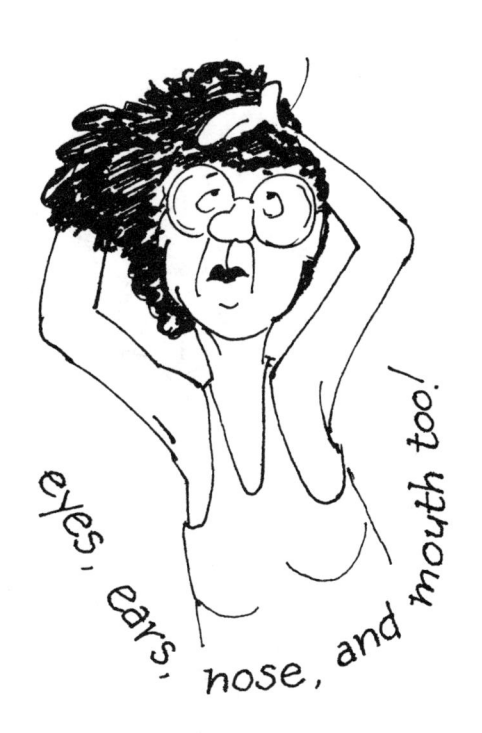

eyes, ears, nose, and mouth too!

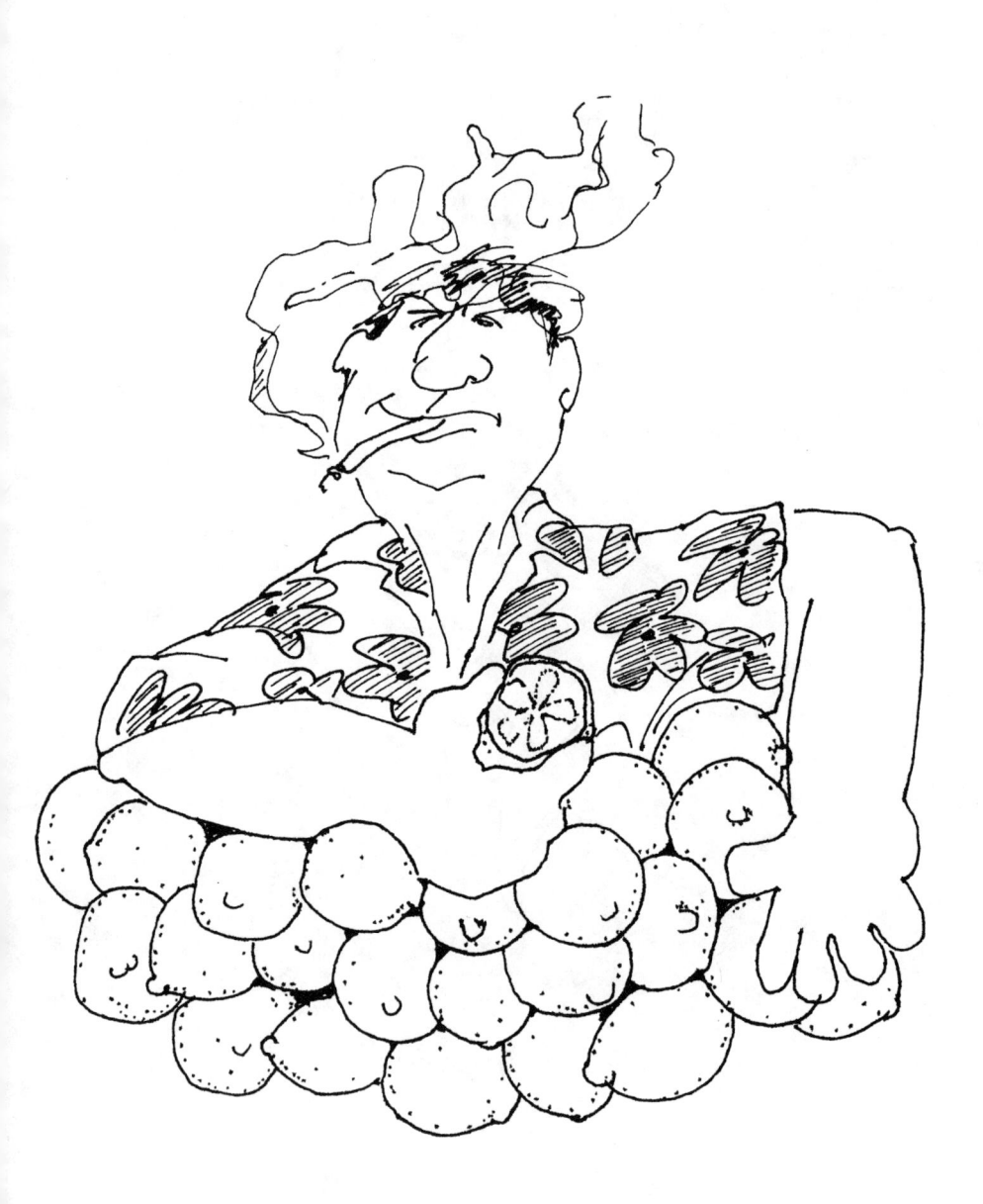

A drop of lemon juice in a little water can be used as eyedrops for irritated eyes.

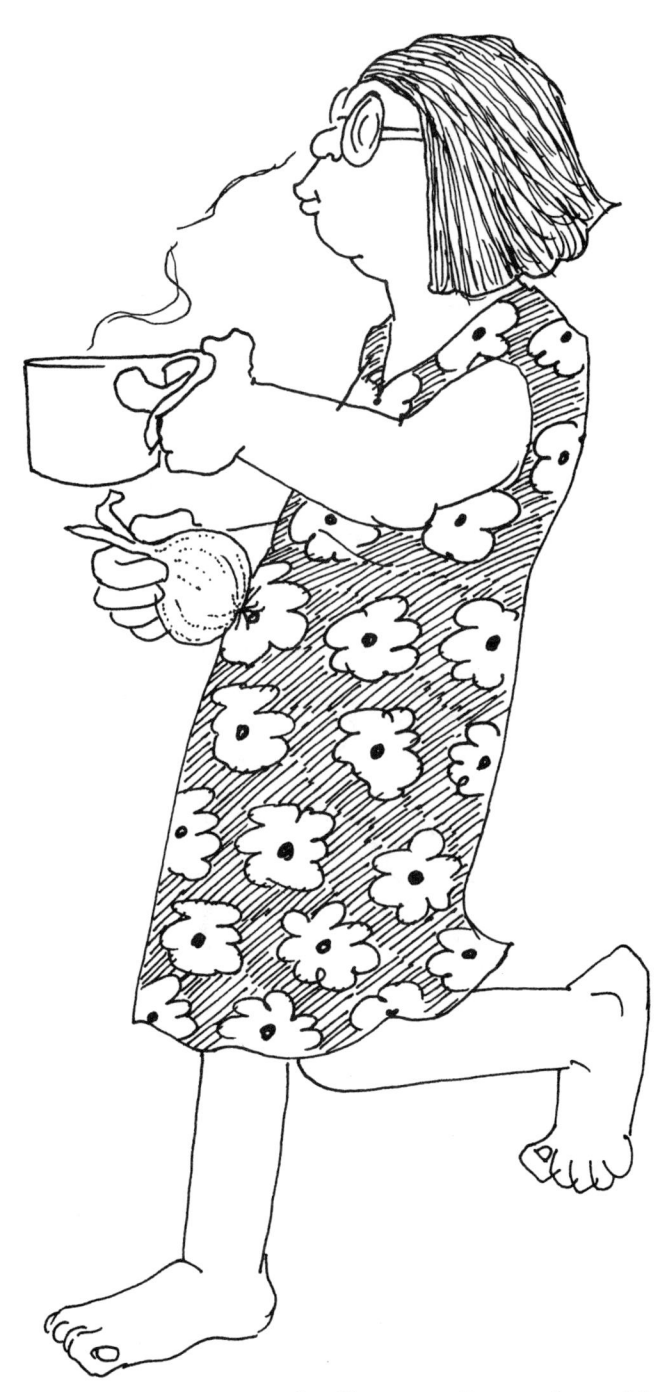

To strengthen weak eyes, boil some dry onion skin in water. Strain the "tea" and drink a cup every day.

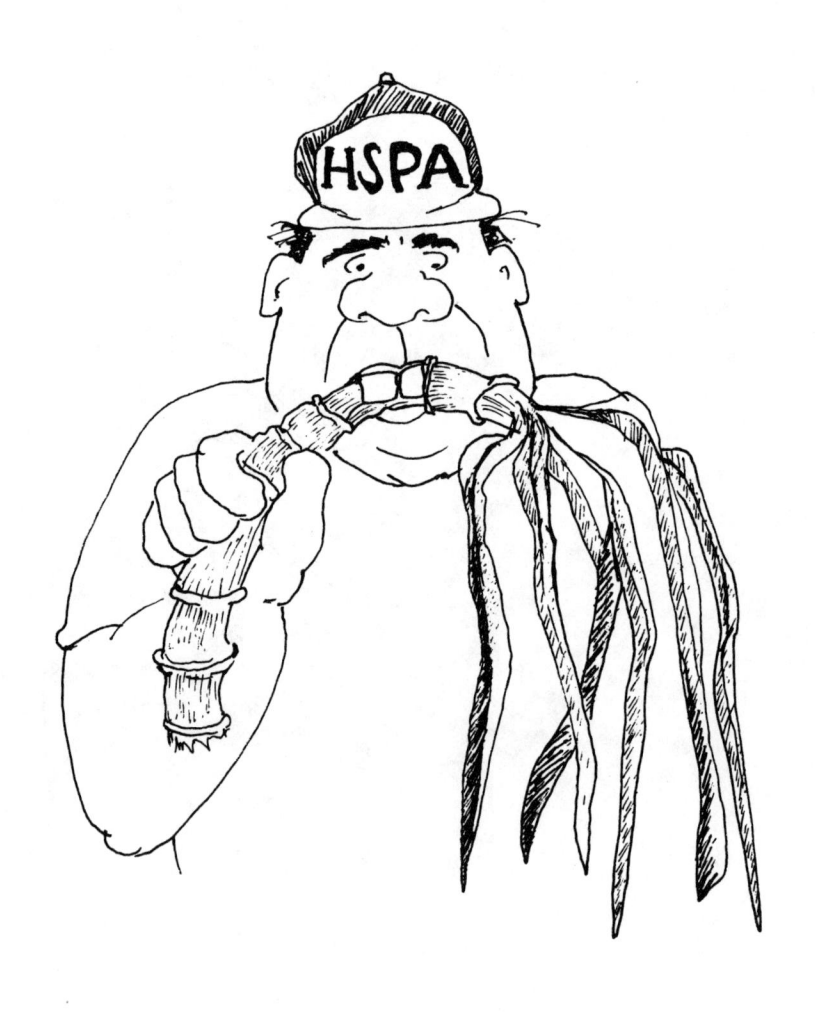

Chew sugar cane to strengthen teeth and gums.

For toothaches, take a partially cooked piece of wild ginger, shape it to cover the aching tooth and bite down on it.

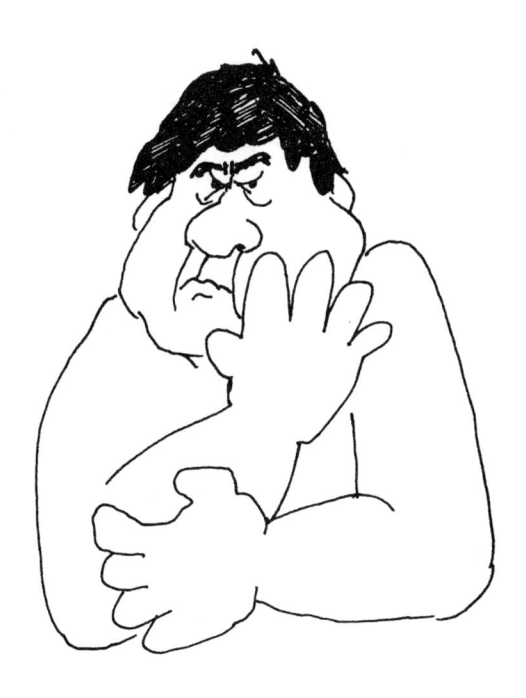

Pua-kala, or Hawaiian poppy root, chewed and inserted into a cavity, will stop toothaches.

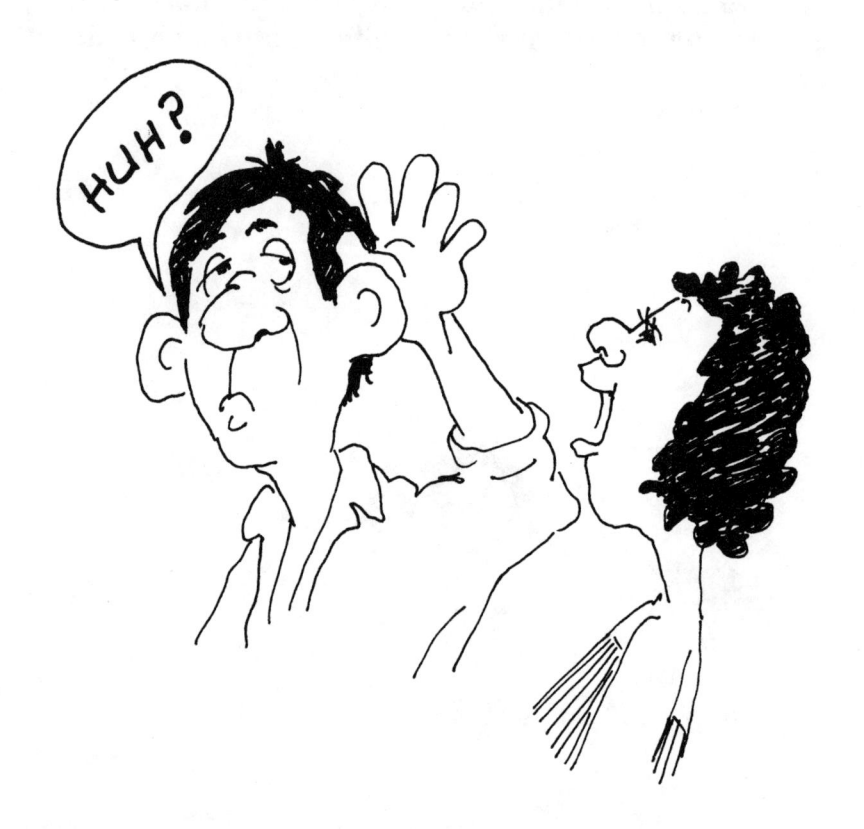

Onion juice dropped into the ear will cure deafness.

For earaches, pound 'olena root, put it in a thin cloth, heat it, and squeeze the juice into the ear.

A few drops of urine in the ear will cure an earache.

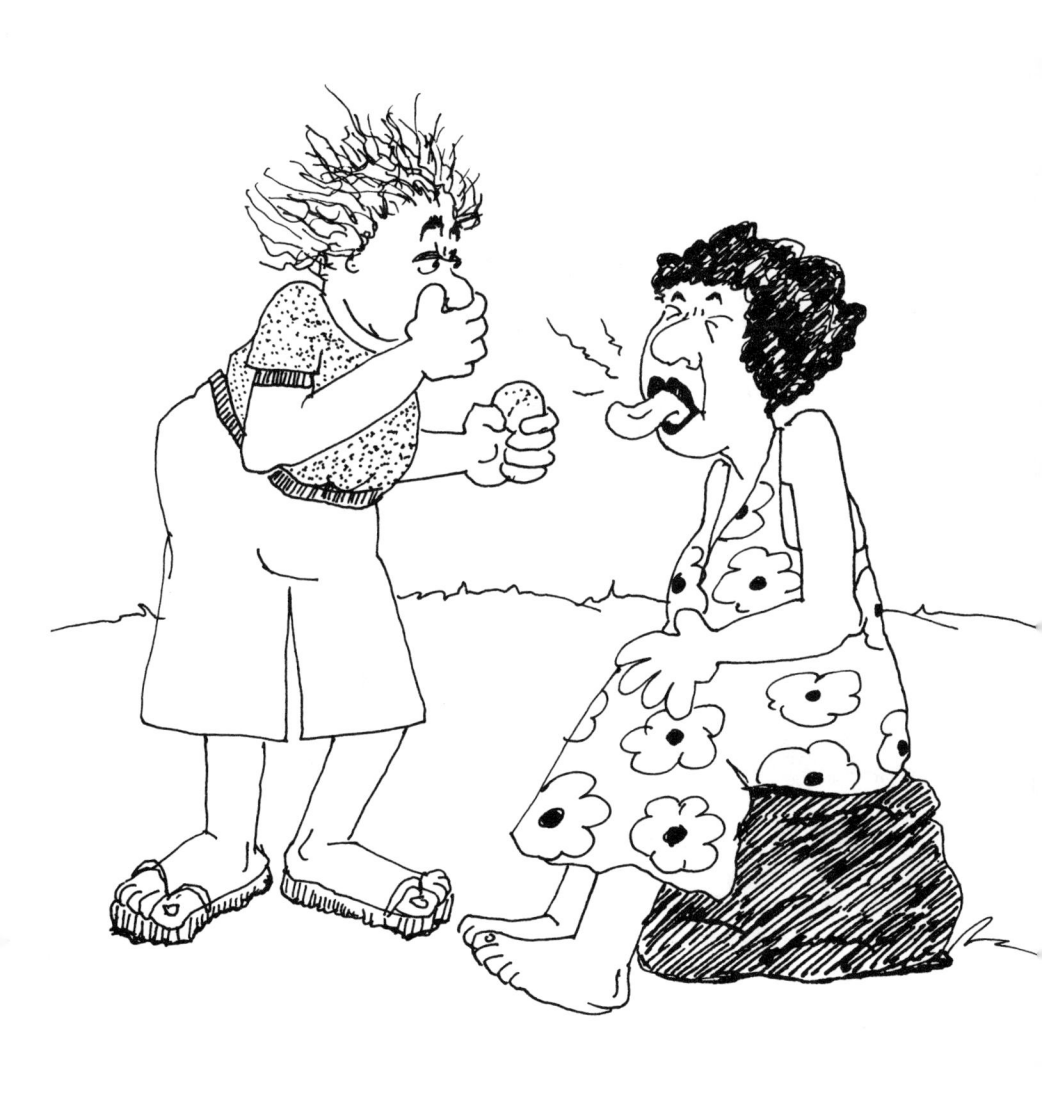

To get rid of bad breath rub the watery sap from a green kukui nut on your tongue.

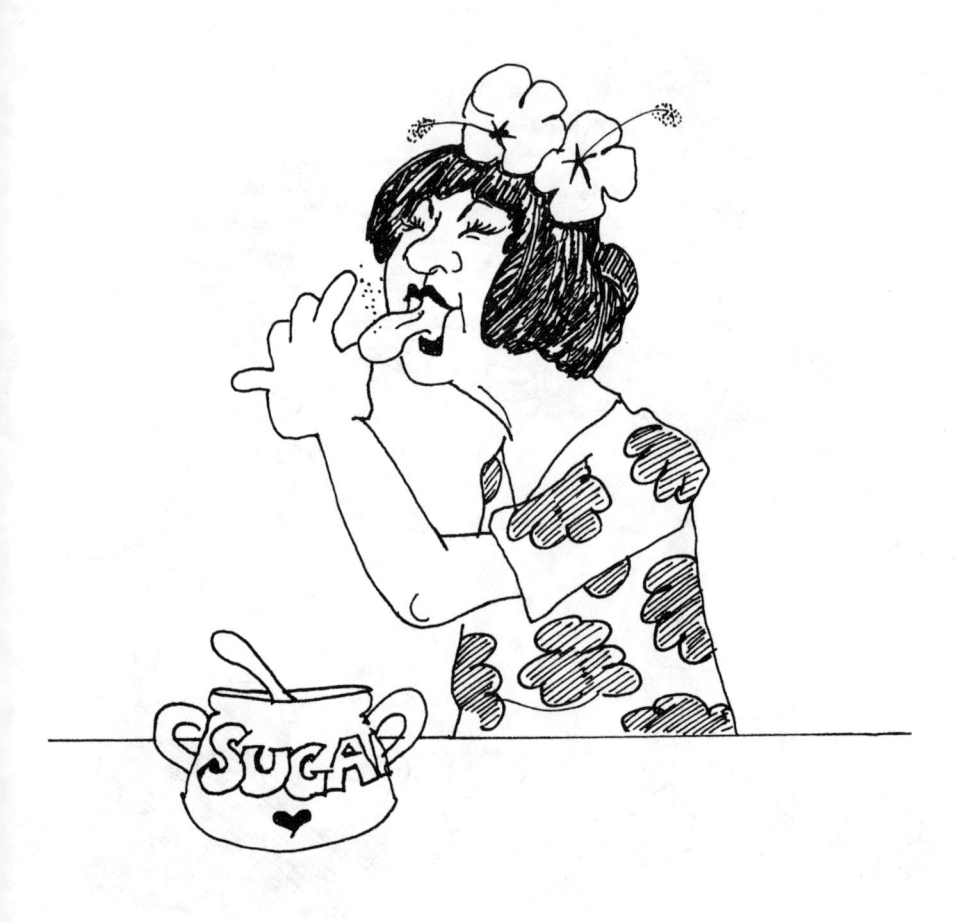

Sprinkle some sugar on your tongue if you burn it with hot food.

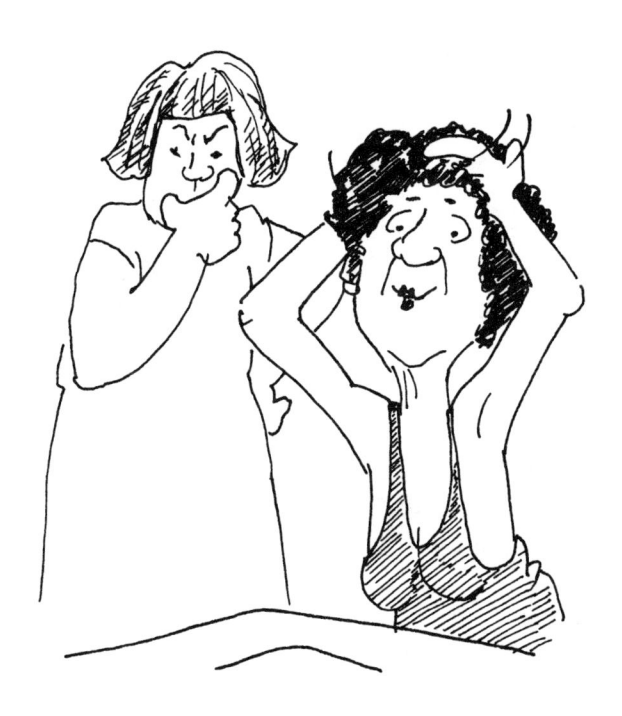

Boil garlic stems in water and wash your hair with the garlic water to get rid of dandruff.

To get rid of ukus (head lice), mash 5 noni fruit, squeeze out the juice, and rub it into the head.

Crushed leaves and bark of the sandalwood tree mixed with hot water kills ukus and gets rid of dandruff. The application should be made 3 times a day for 3 successive days.

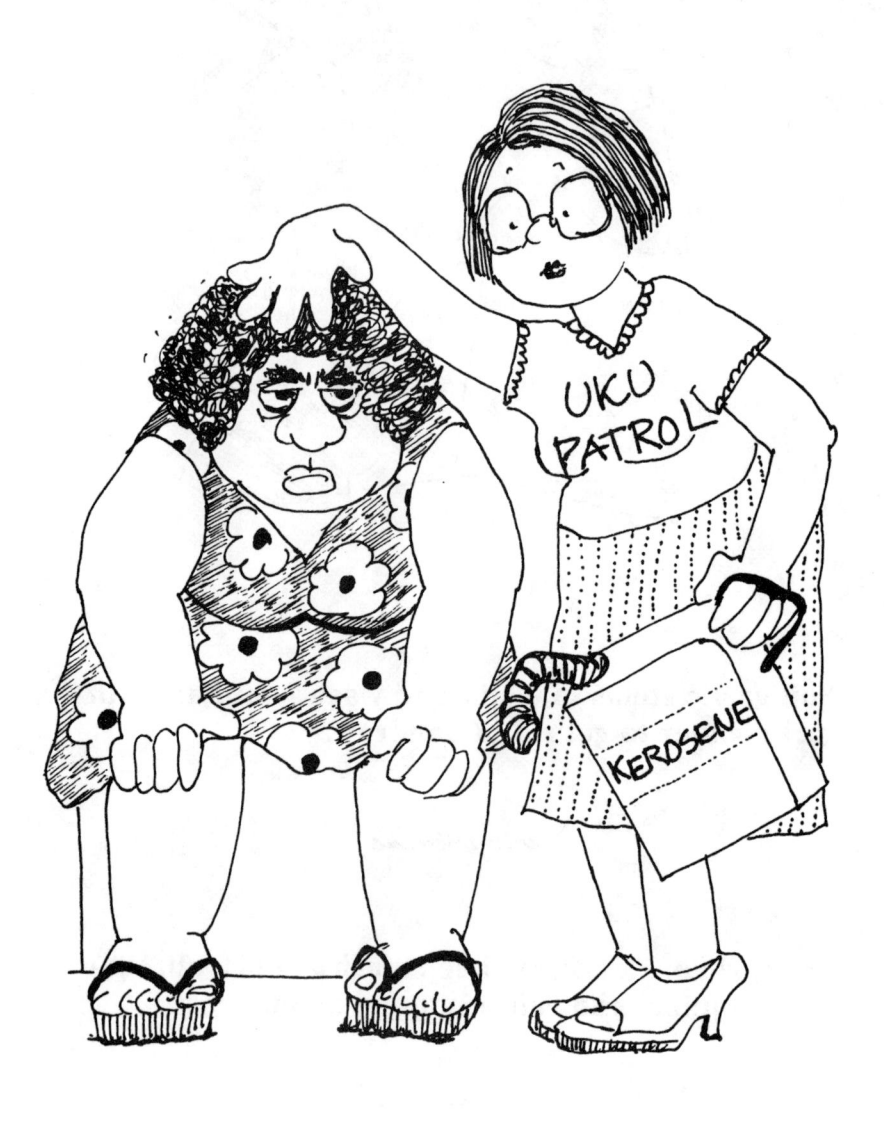

Rub kerosene into the hair to get rid of ukus.

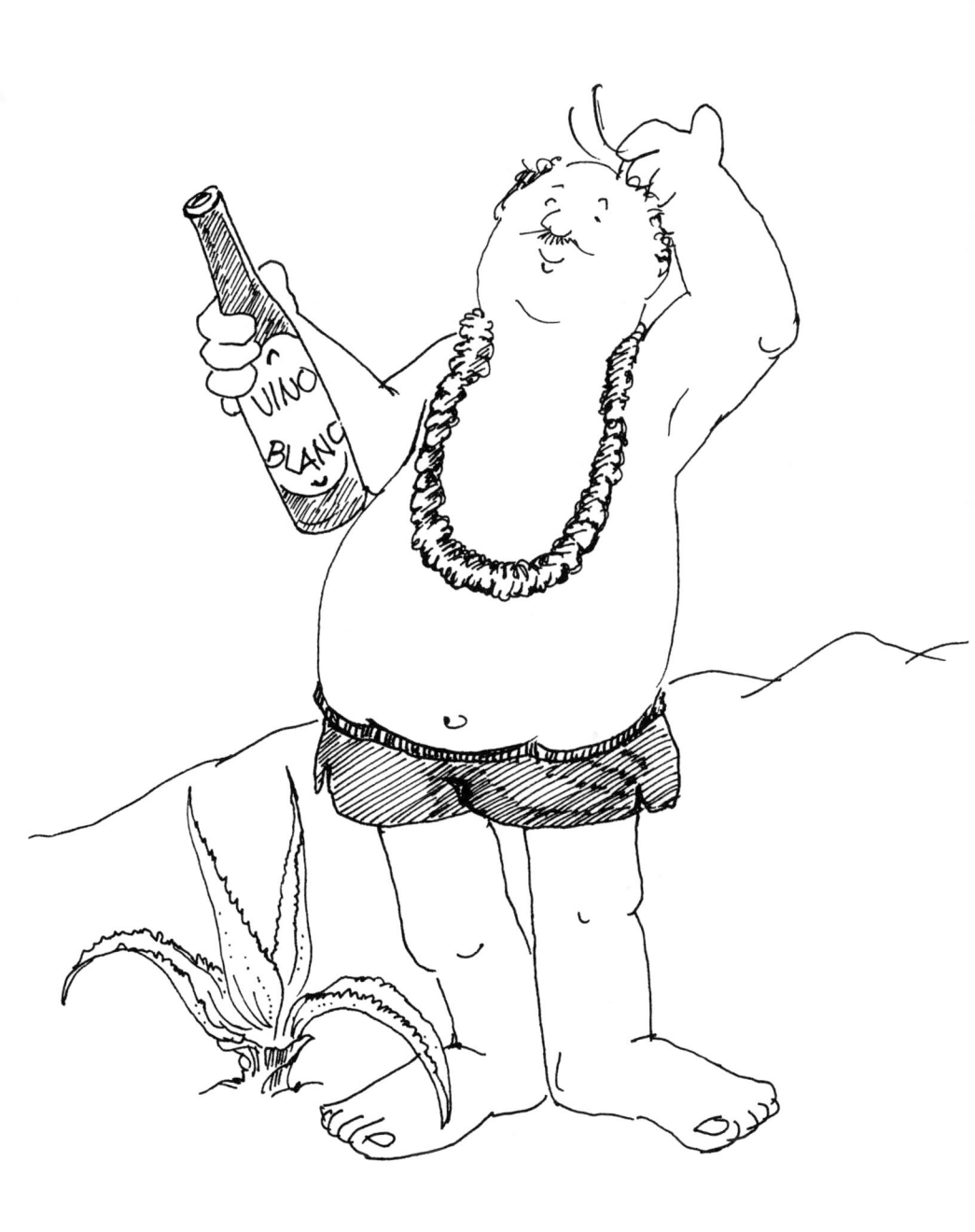

To prevent hair loss, combine the juice of aloe with some wine and rub the mixture into your scalp.

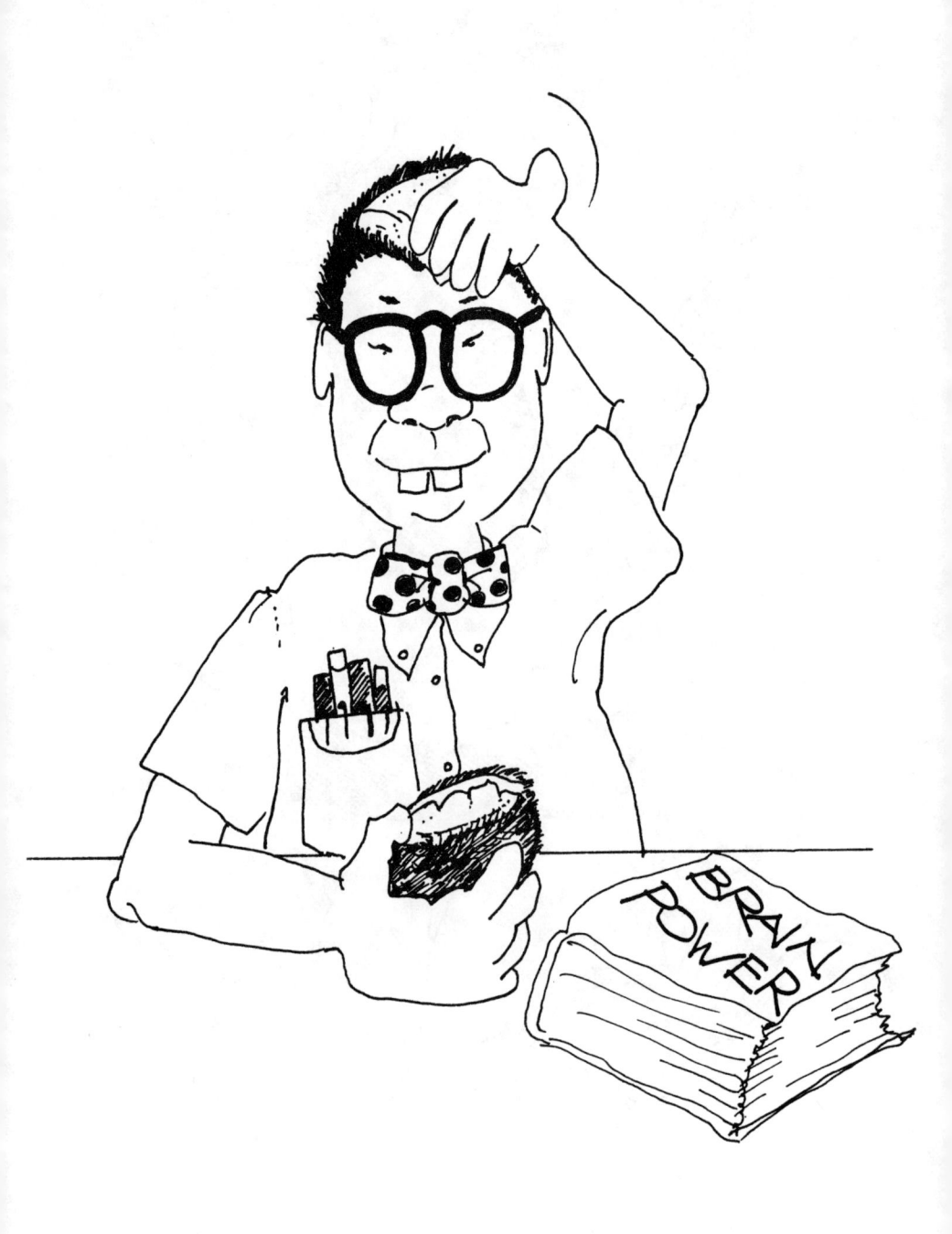

The meat of a young coconut is good for the brain . . . rub it on your head.

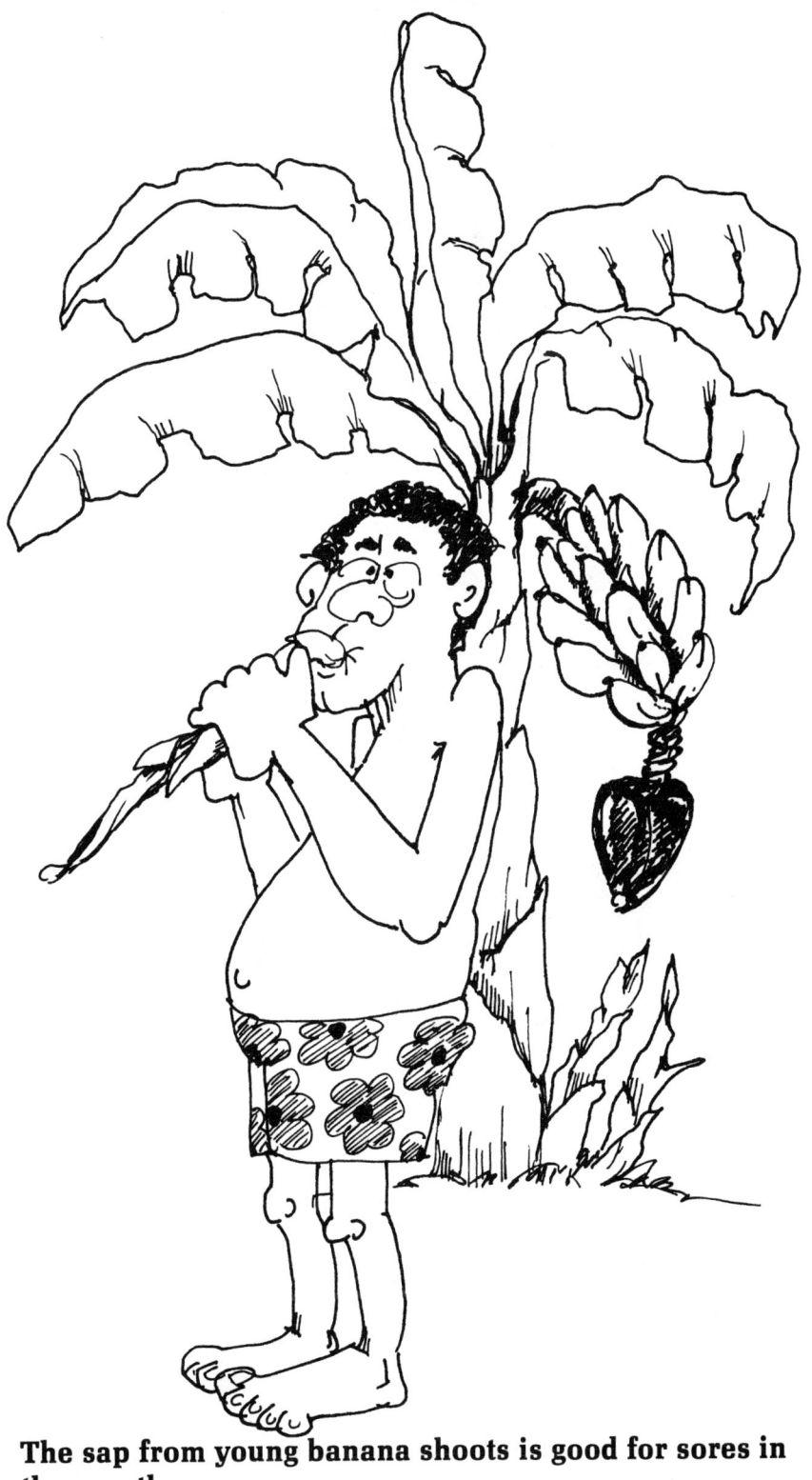

The sap from young banana shoots is good for sores in the mouth.

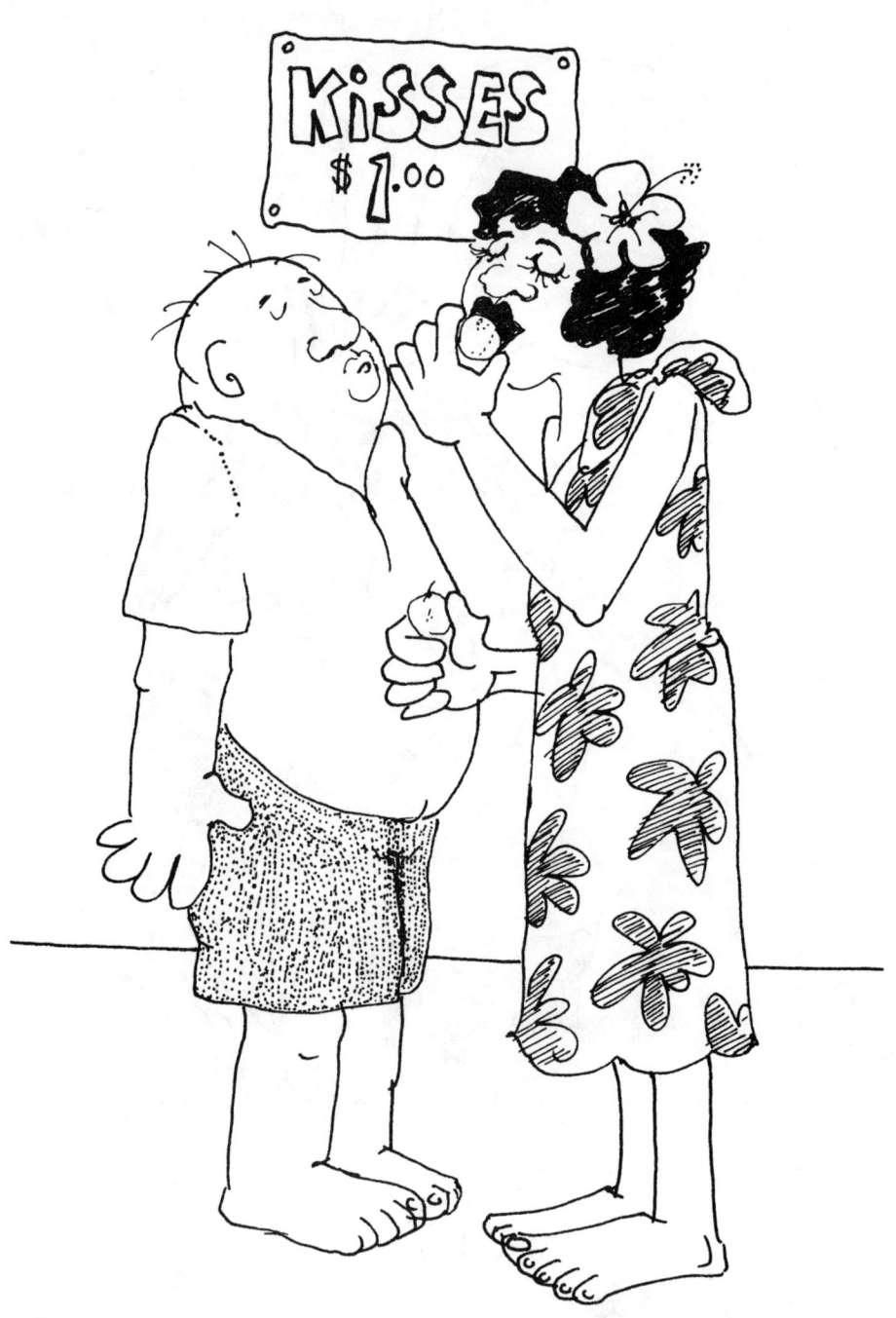

For chapped lips, pull the stem off a kukui nut. Rub the sap that oozes out of the "well" left by the stem on your lips.

Stomach Problems

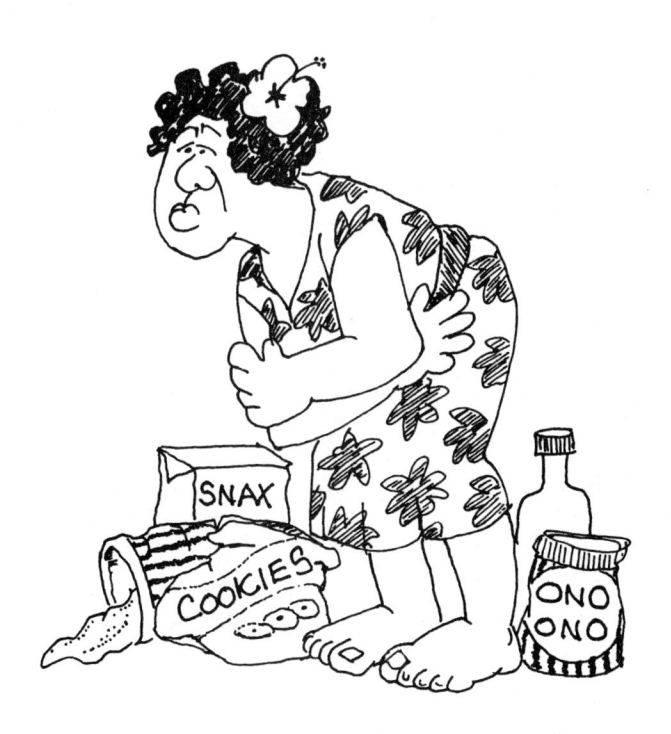

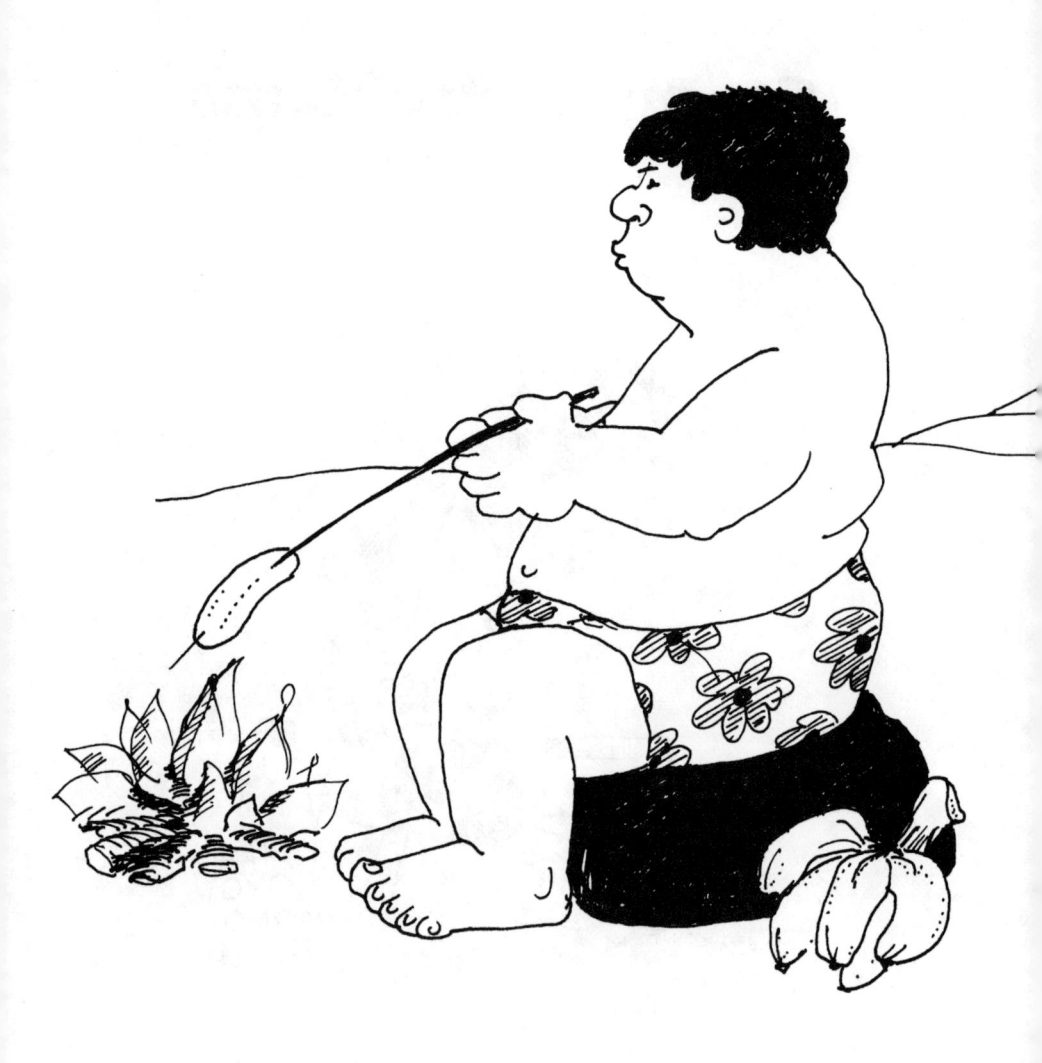

To end diarrhea, peel a green banana, broil it over a fire, and eat it.

Drink tea made out of guava leaf buds to relieve diarrhea.

Ginseng tonic relieves indigestion, vomiting, and diarrhea.

Make a tea out of dried pomegranate rind by simmering it in hot water. Drink a small cup of it to relieve stomach ache and diarrhea.

A spoonful of pia (arrowroot) starch in a small amount of poi will cure diarrhea.

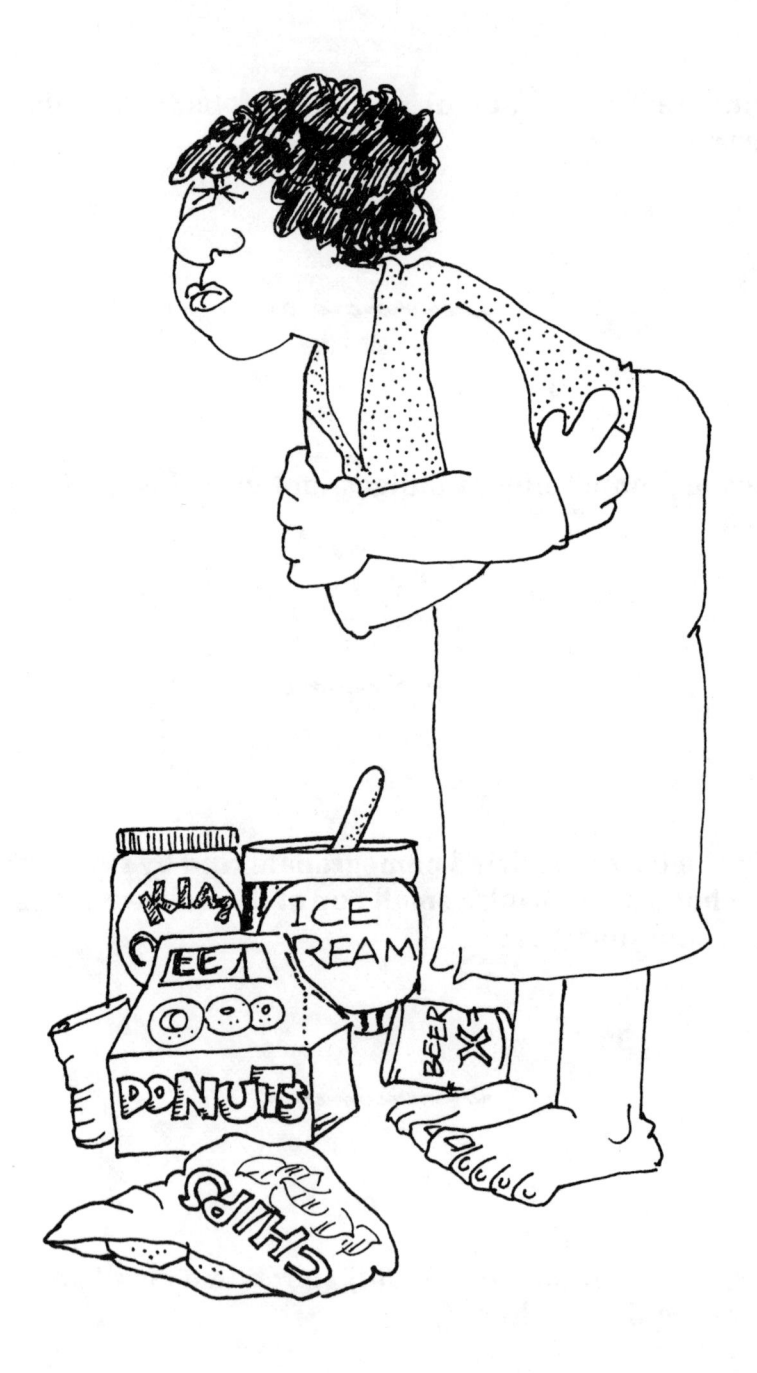

Pound the leaves of yomogi (mugwort) and drink the juice obtained from them to relieve stomach cramps.

To relieve constipation, boil aloe leaves (about 5 ounces) in 2 cups of water until the liquid is reduced to ½ cup. Strain and drink the juice before you go to bed at night.

Chewing the soft part at the base of hala flowers will cure constipation.

Chew the base of hibiscus buds to relieve constipation.

The oil of kukui nuts makes a potent laxative.

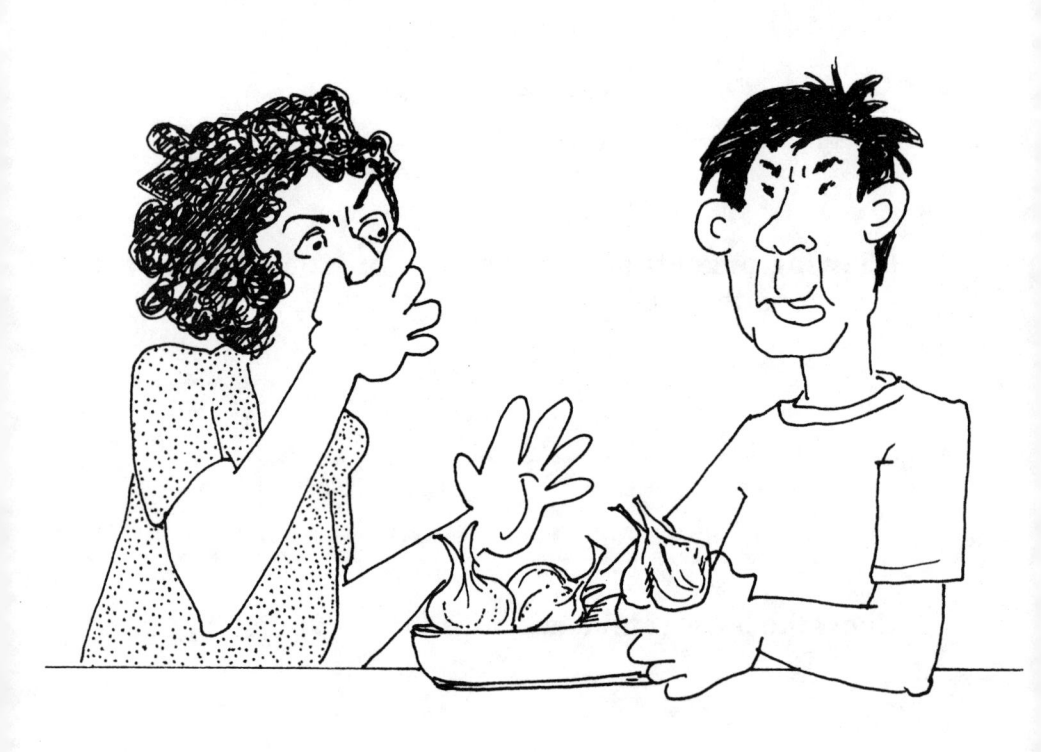

Eat raw garlic to cure stomach ulcers.

For bleeding ulcers, pound 'olena root, squeeze the juice out of it, and drink 1 tablespoon 2 times a day.

Bleeding from the bowels can be treated in the following way: Pound together 3 guava roots, 2 shoots of the hala tree, and a handful of Chinese banana roots. Cook in some water and strain the liquid. Drink a mouthful of the mixture several times a day.

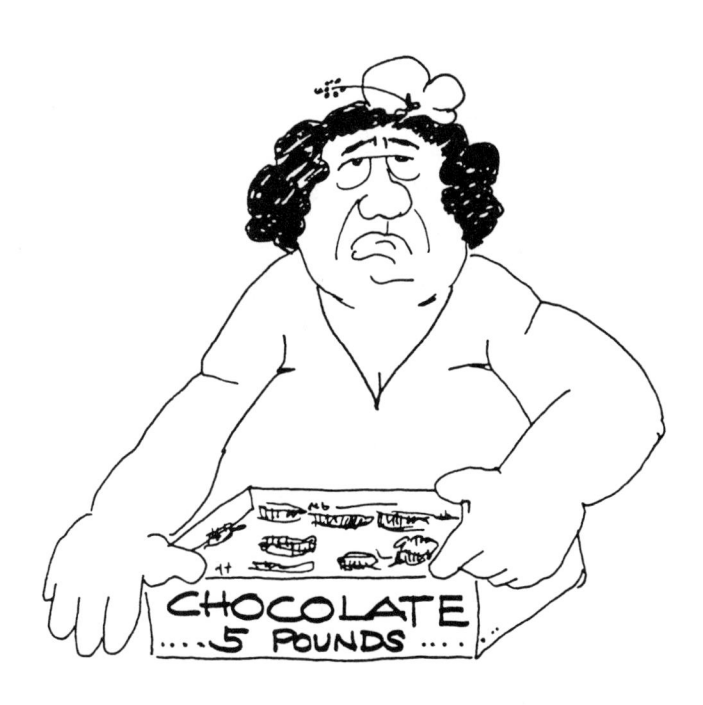

To induce vomiting (because a person has eaten something bad or too much), scrape a raw sweet potato and a ti leaf stem. Add water, and place in the sun. Strain the mixture and drink it.

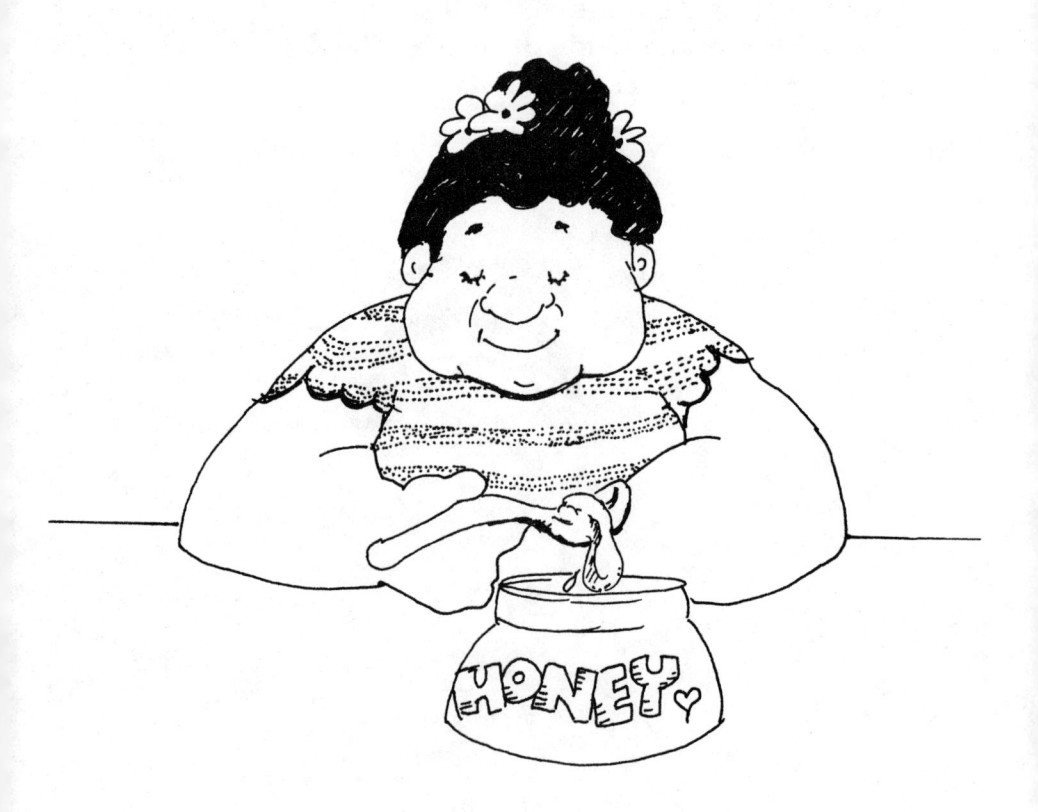

To ease the pain of stomach ulcers, eat an ounce of honey before each meal.

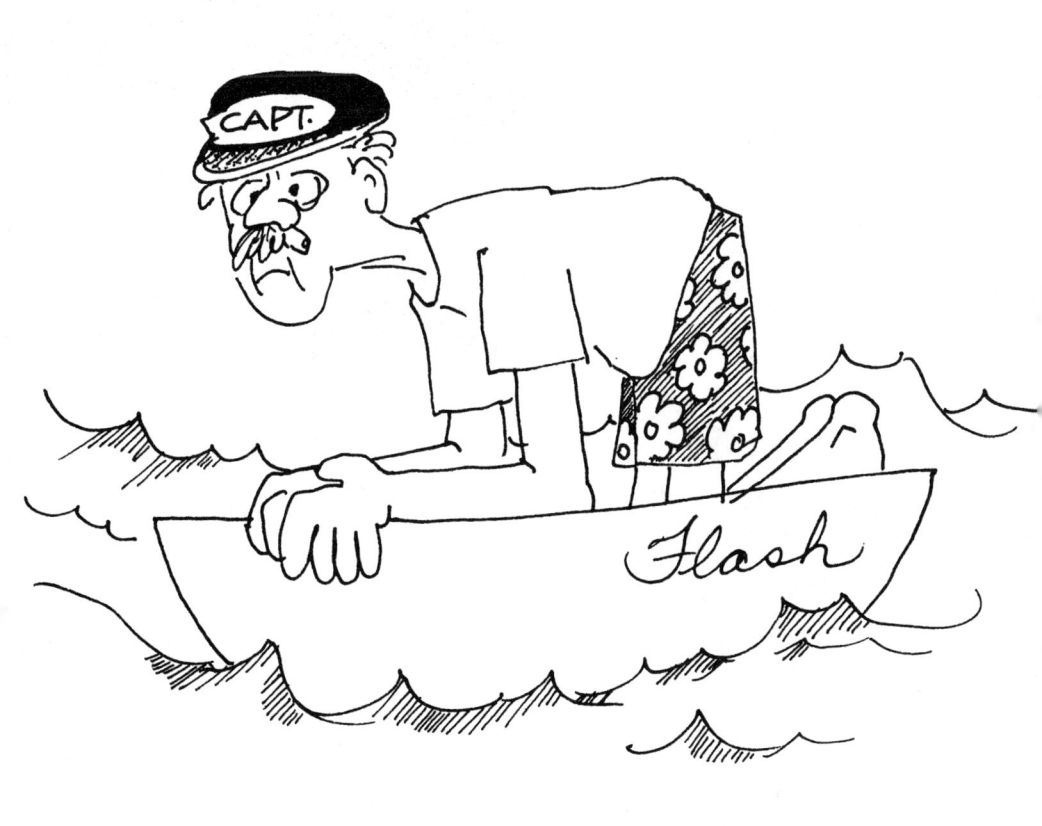

Chinese ginger is good for seasickness. Chew a small piece of ginger (candied or preserved ginger is good) during a boat ride.

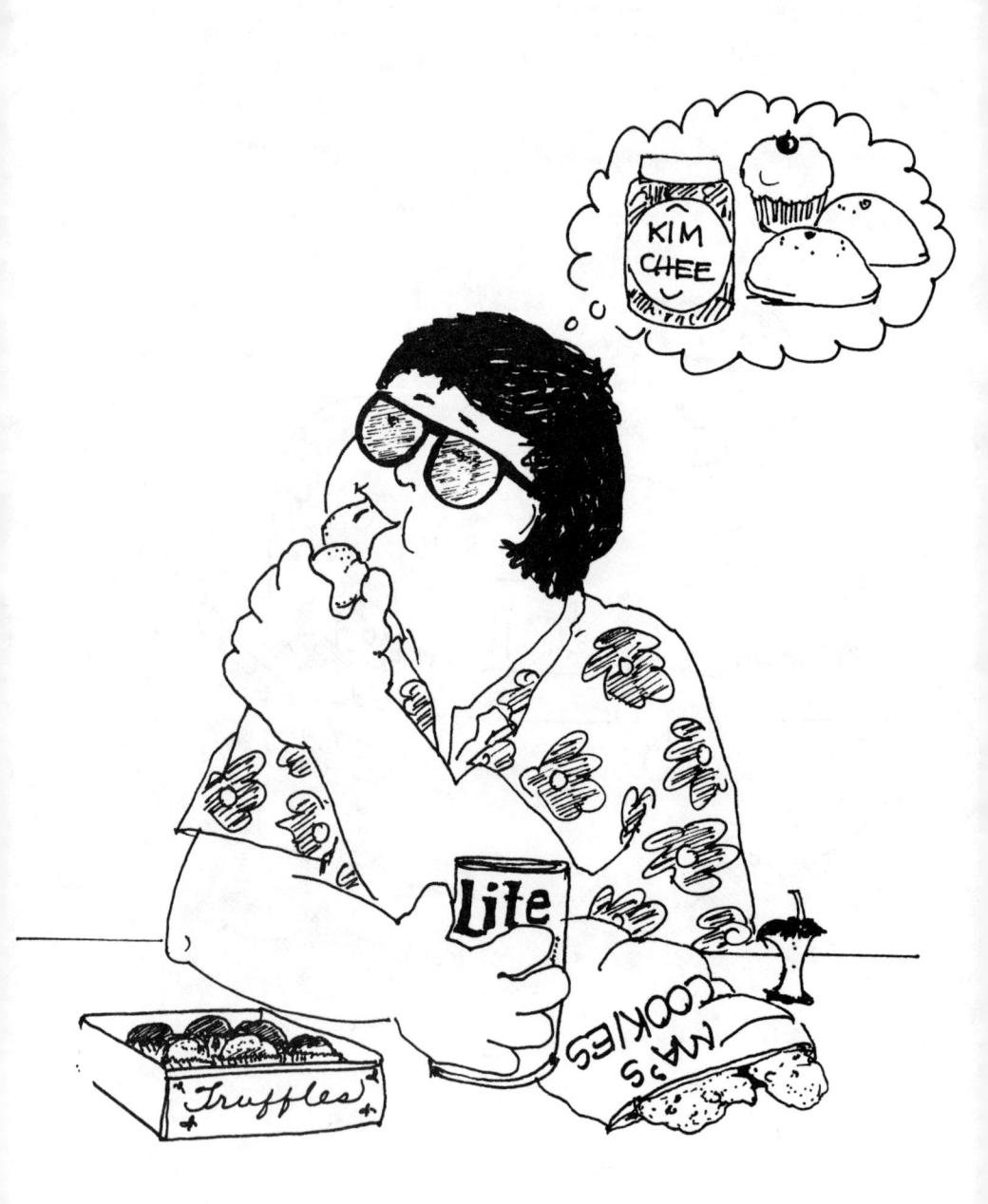

To soothe an upset stomach, break the stem off a kukui nut and lick the sap which oozes off the nut.

Eat okai (rice gruel) and ume (Japanese pickled plum) when you feel nauseous. The rice soothes the stomach and ume acts as an antacid.

For intestinal disorders, eat dry seeds of laukāhi (about 1 teaspoon twice a day).

Eating papaya helps people with digestive problems.

To treat indigestion, take about 2 inches of Chinese ginger root, simmer it in water, and drink the tea with each meal.

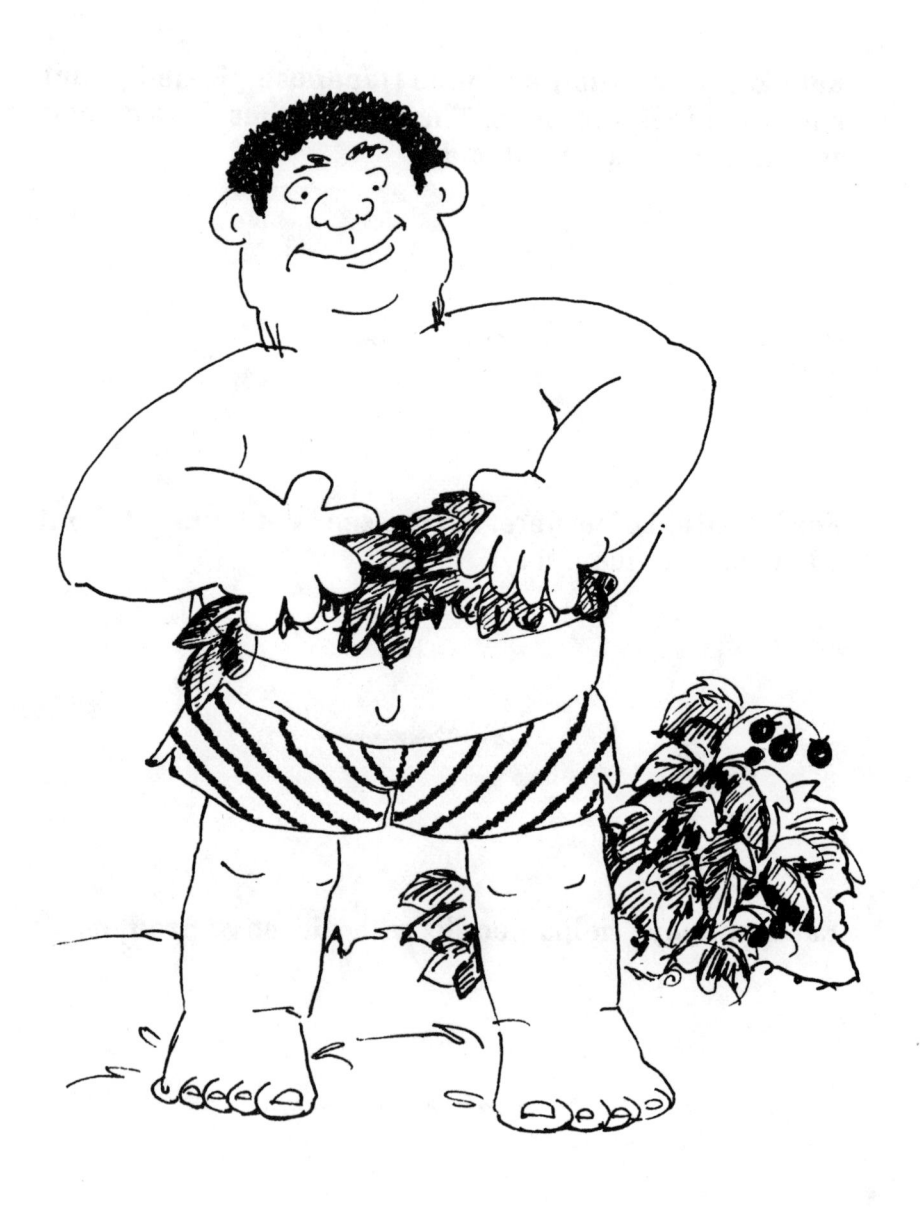

If you have indigestion, gather a bunch of pōpolo leaves and rub them on your ʻōpū.

Other Pilikia

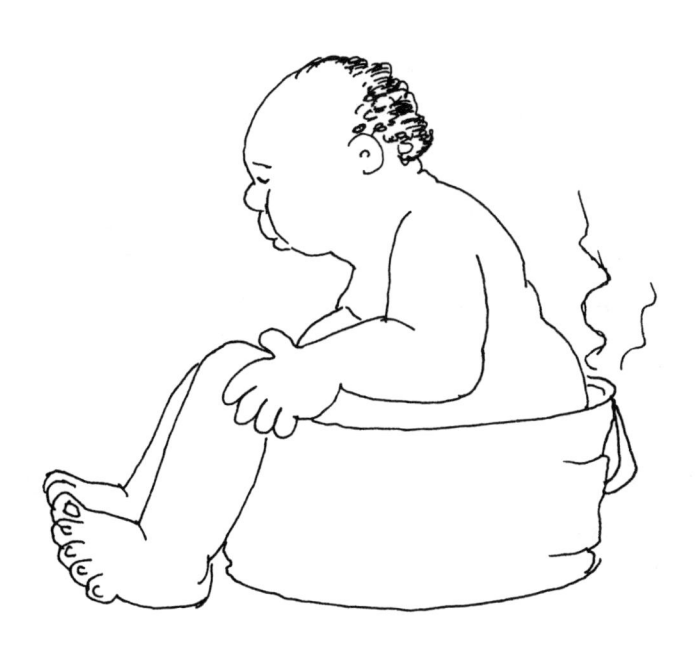

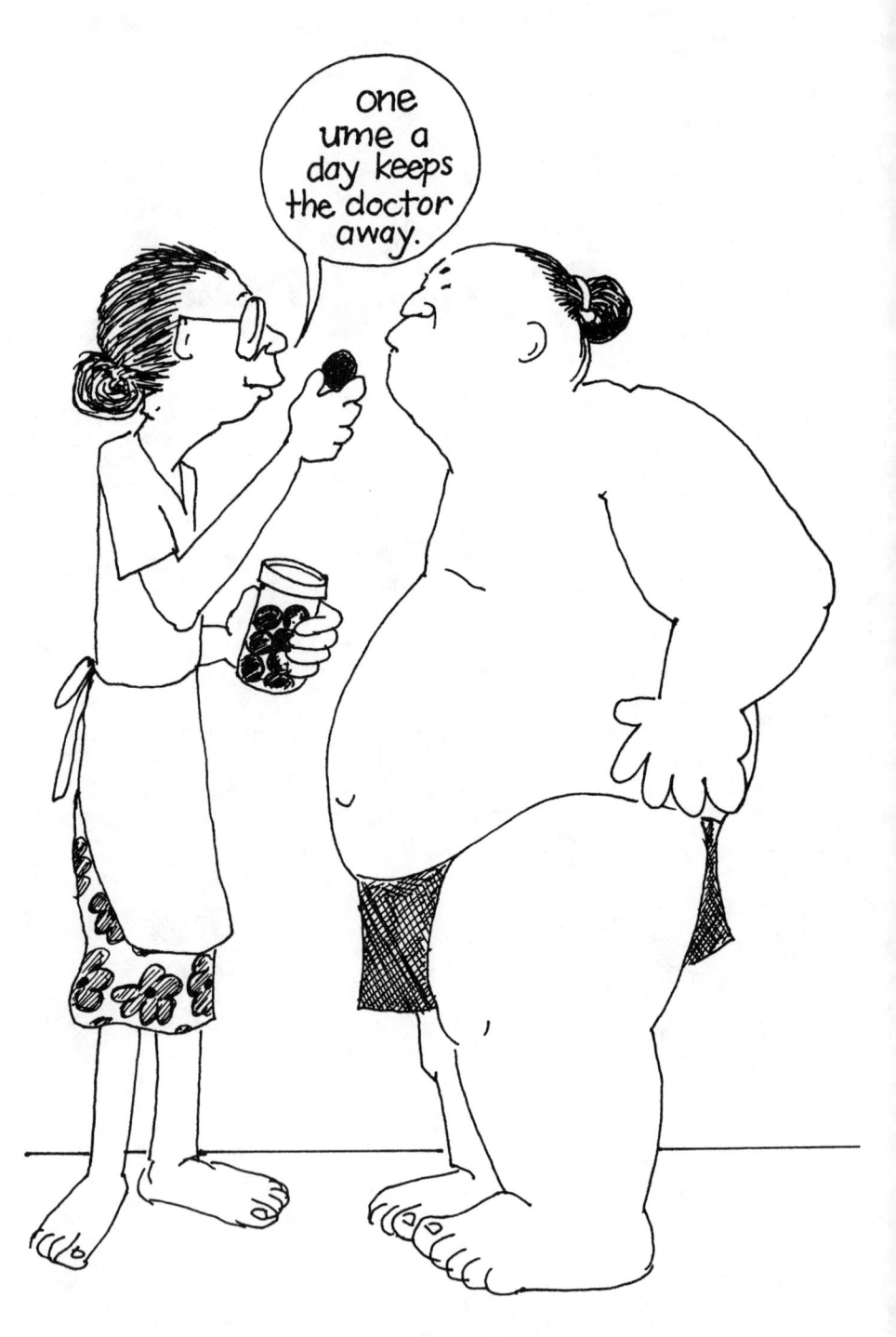

Eat 1 ume a day to keep the body in sound health.

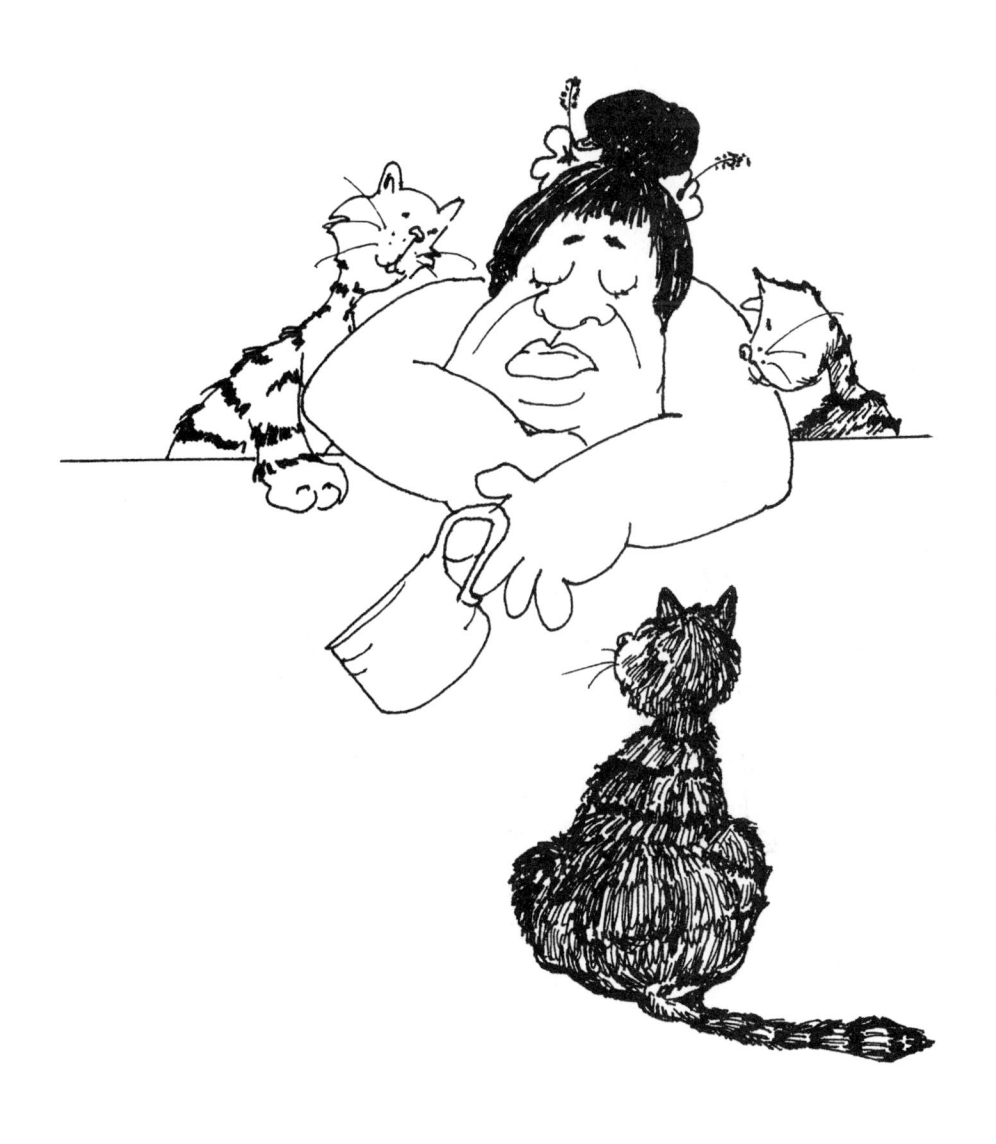

A tea made out of leaves of passion flower helps to induce sleep.

Drink a tea made out of equal parts of chopped ginseng, dried orange peel and a bit of honey to relieve insomnia.

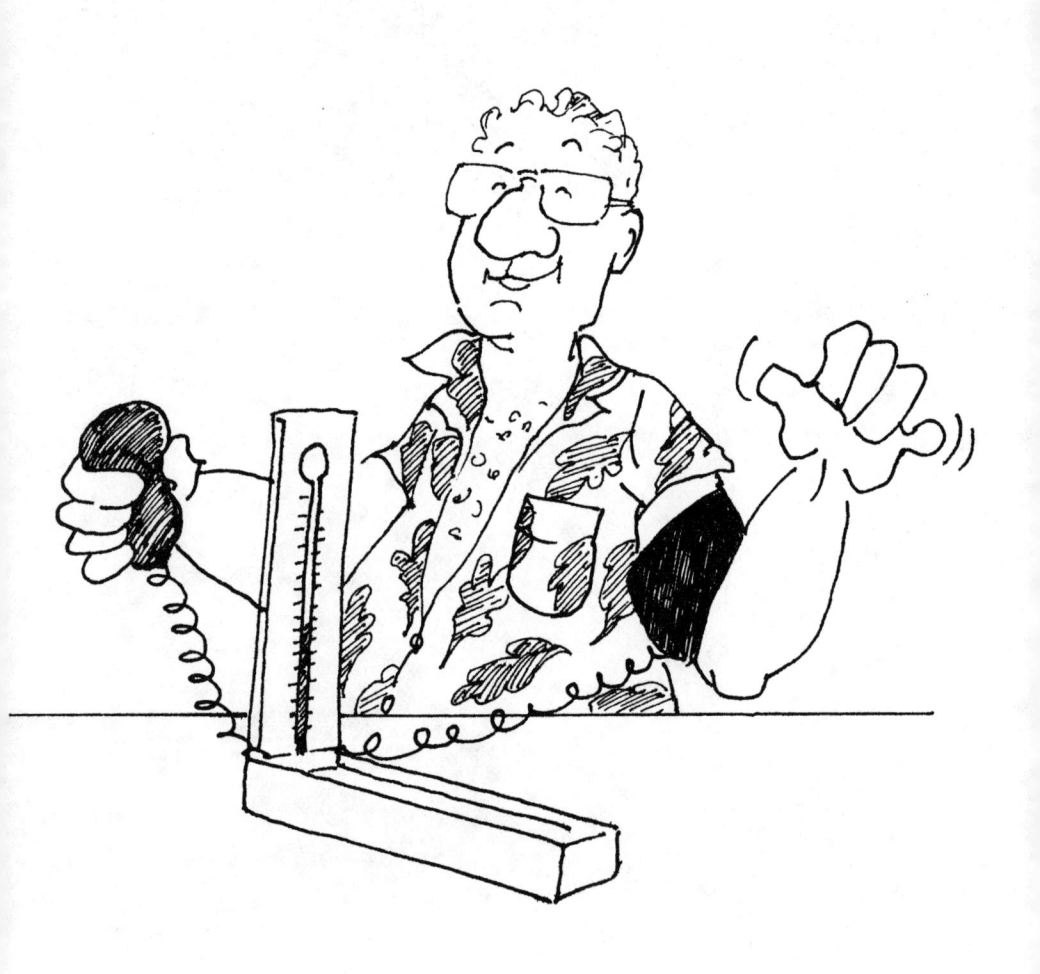

Boil some corn silk in a pint of water until the liquid is reduced by one half. Strain the "tea" and drink it for high blood pressure.

The juice of very ripe noni is good for people with high blood pressure. Crush the fruit, add water to it, and drink it before meals.

Drink tea made out of the leaves of māmaki to reduce high blood pressure.

Make tea out of the buds of Spanish needle and drink it to relieve high blood pressure.

Tea made out of lemon grass is good for high blood pressure.

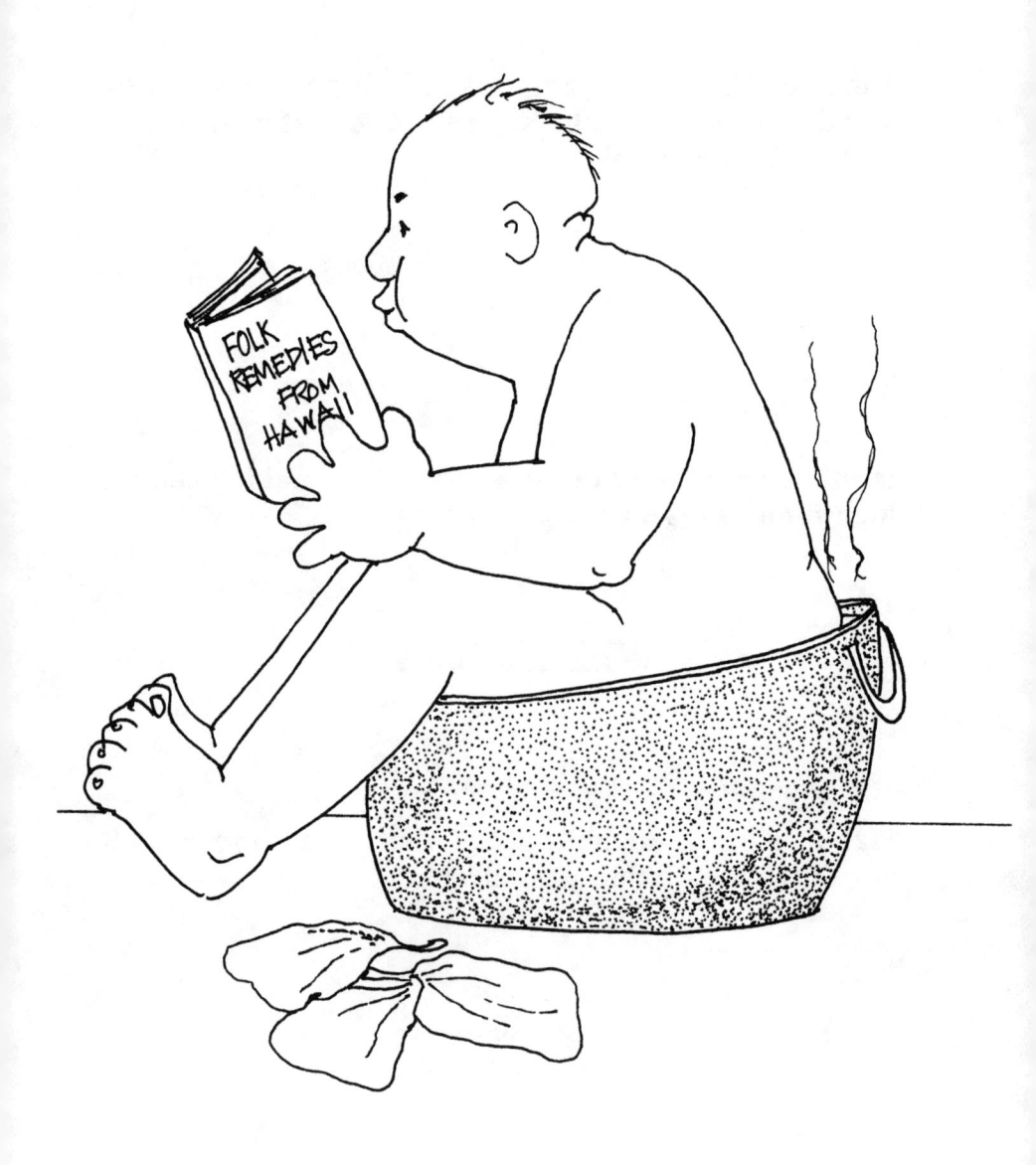

To soothe hemorrhoids, make a brew out of laukāhi leaves and sit in the hot liquid.

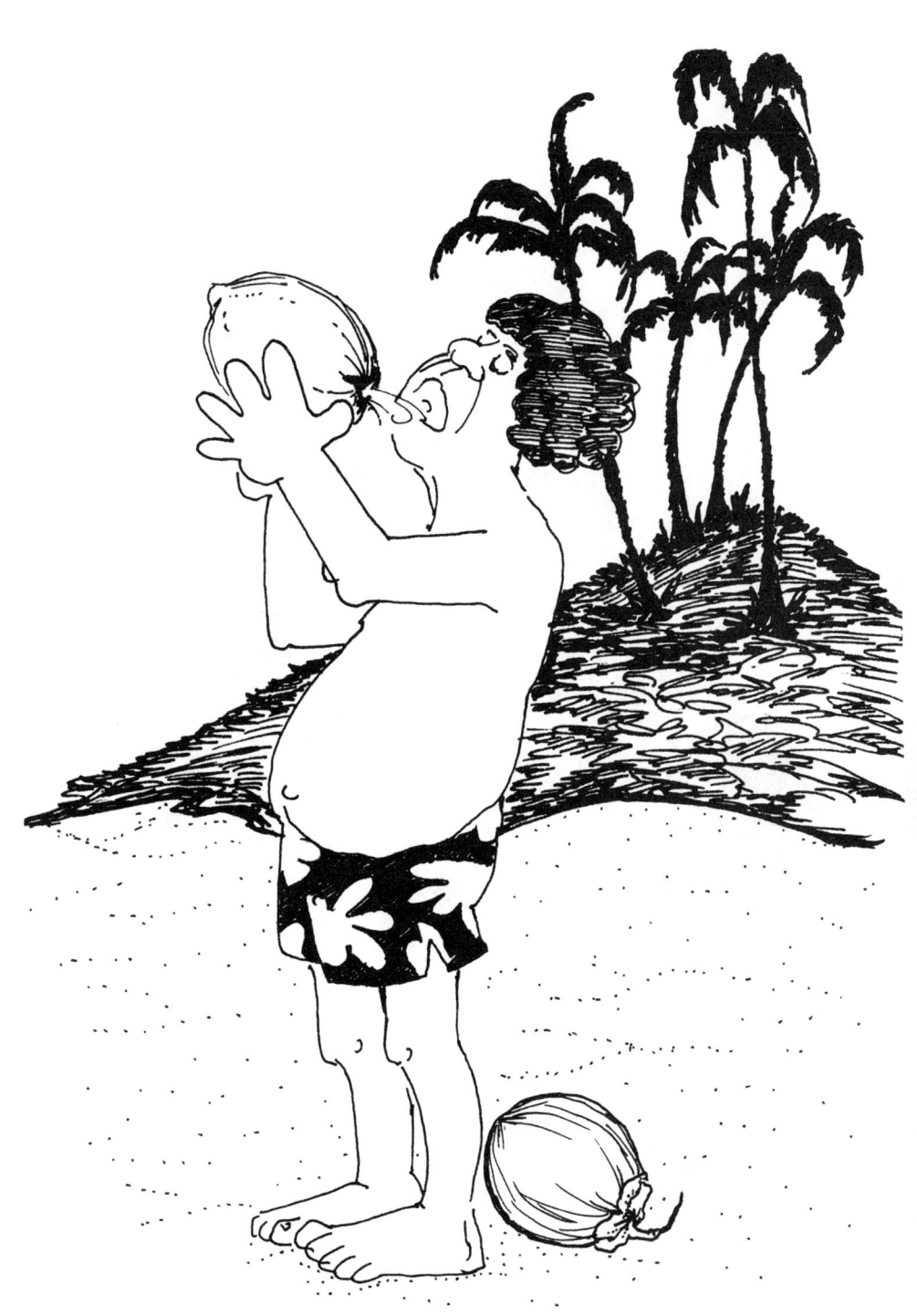

People with kidney problems are helped by drinking coconut water (juice of a fresh coconut) daily.

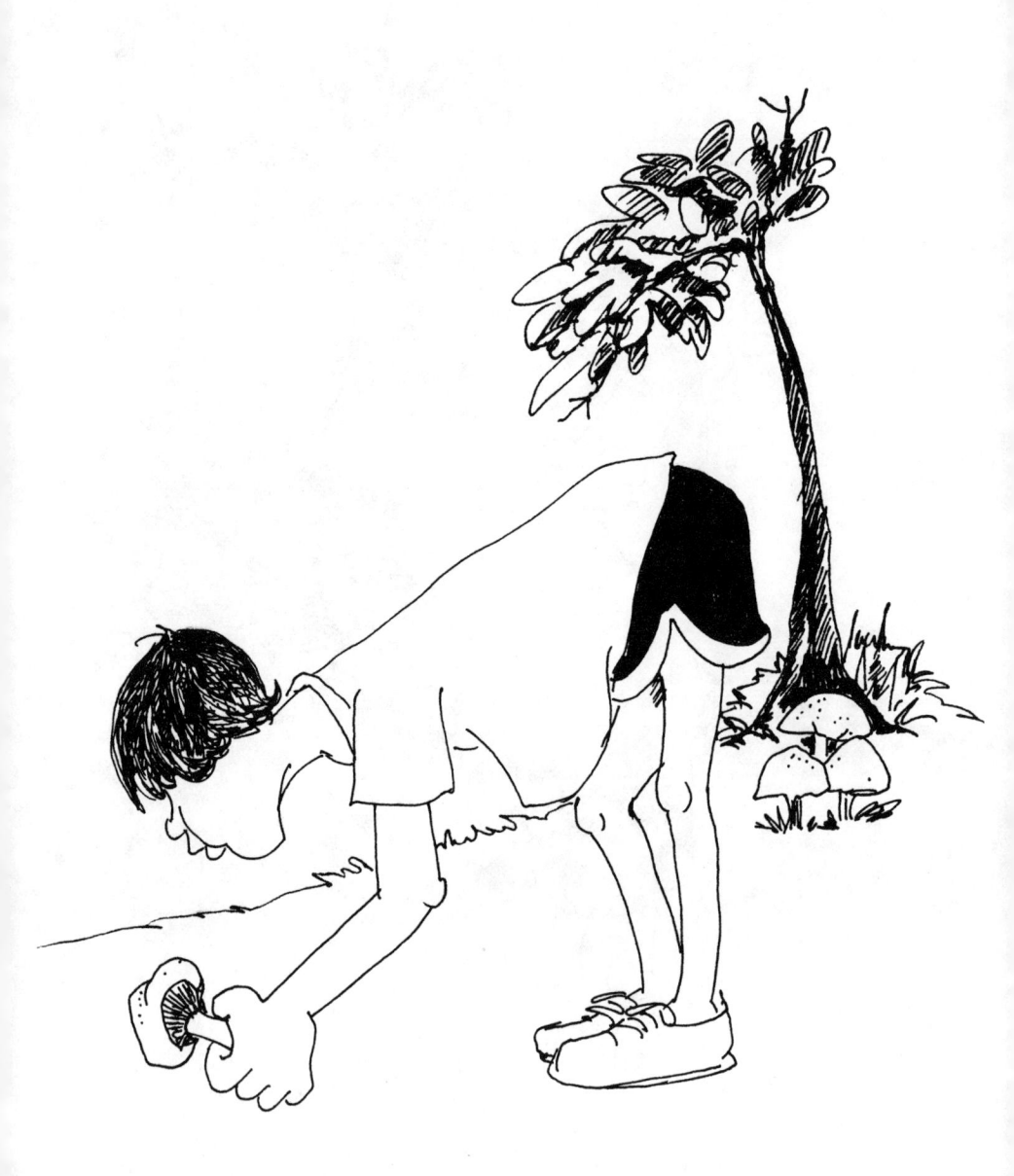

Eating mushrooms and fungi improves memory and strengthens the heart.

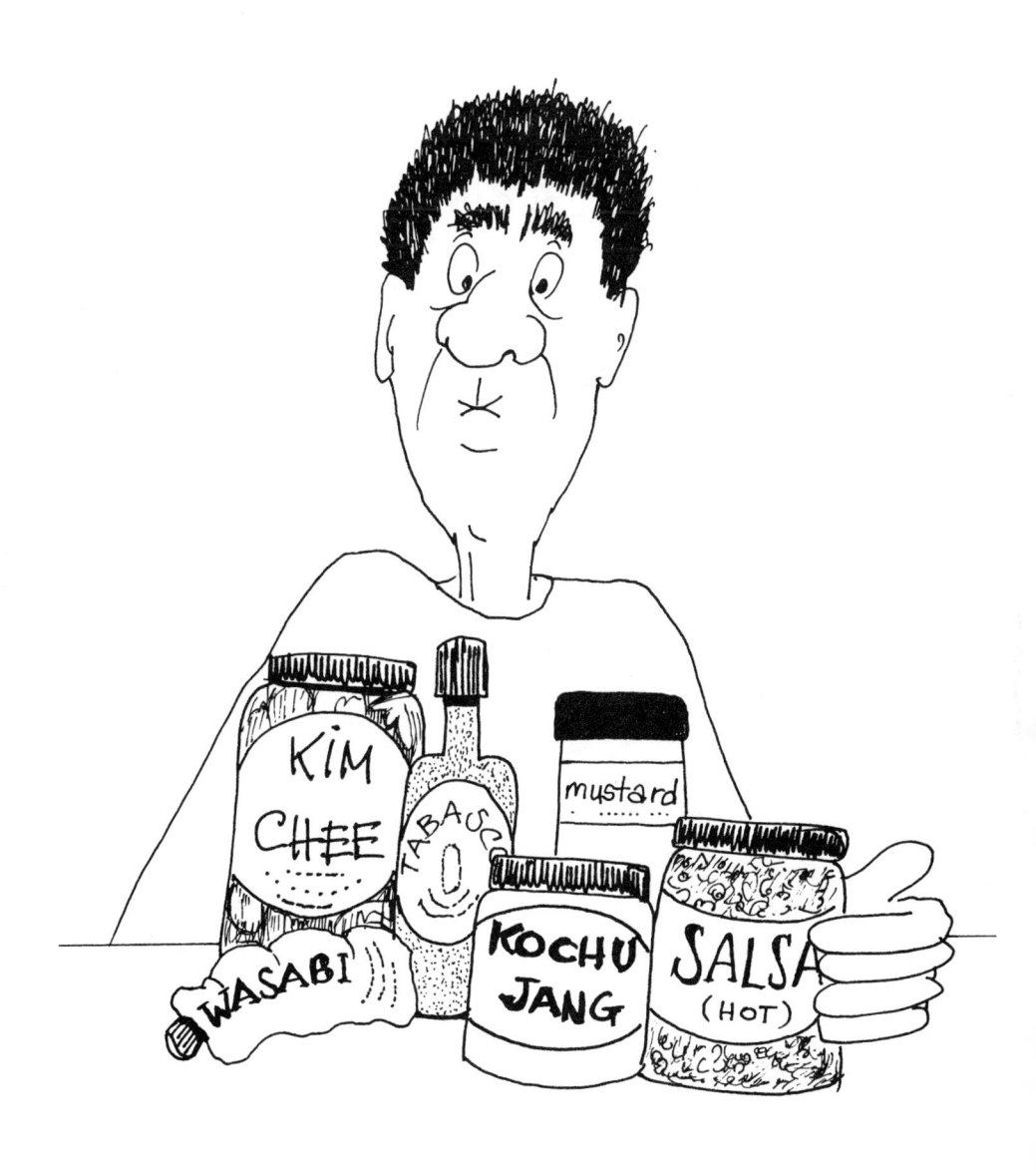

Eating hot, spicy foods helps people with bronchitis and emphysema.

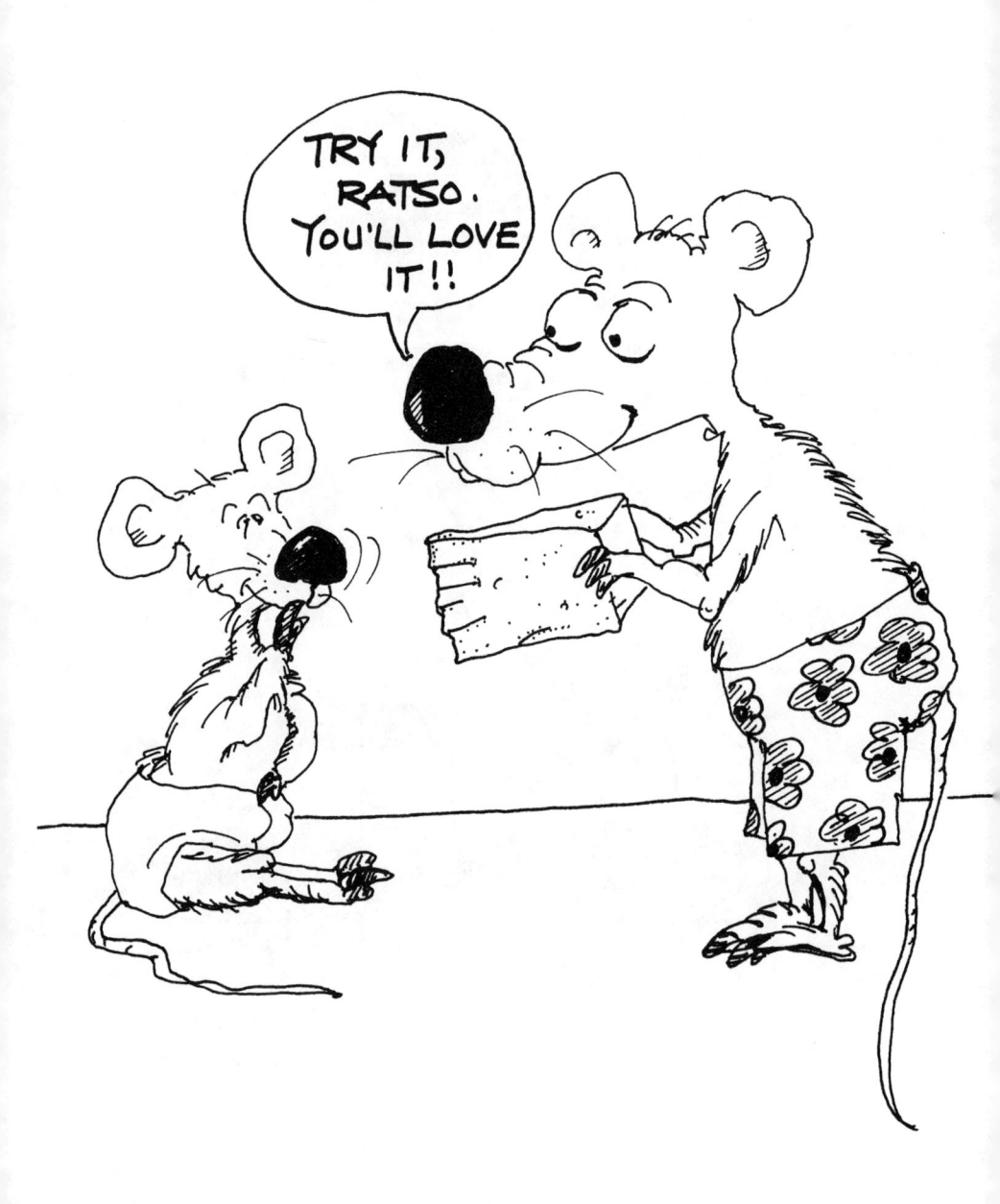

Cheddar cheese helps to relieve asthma.

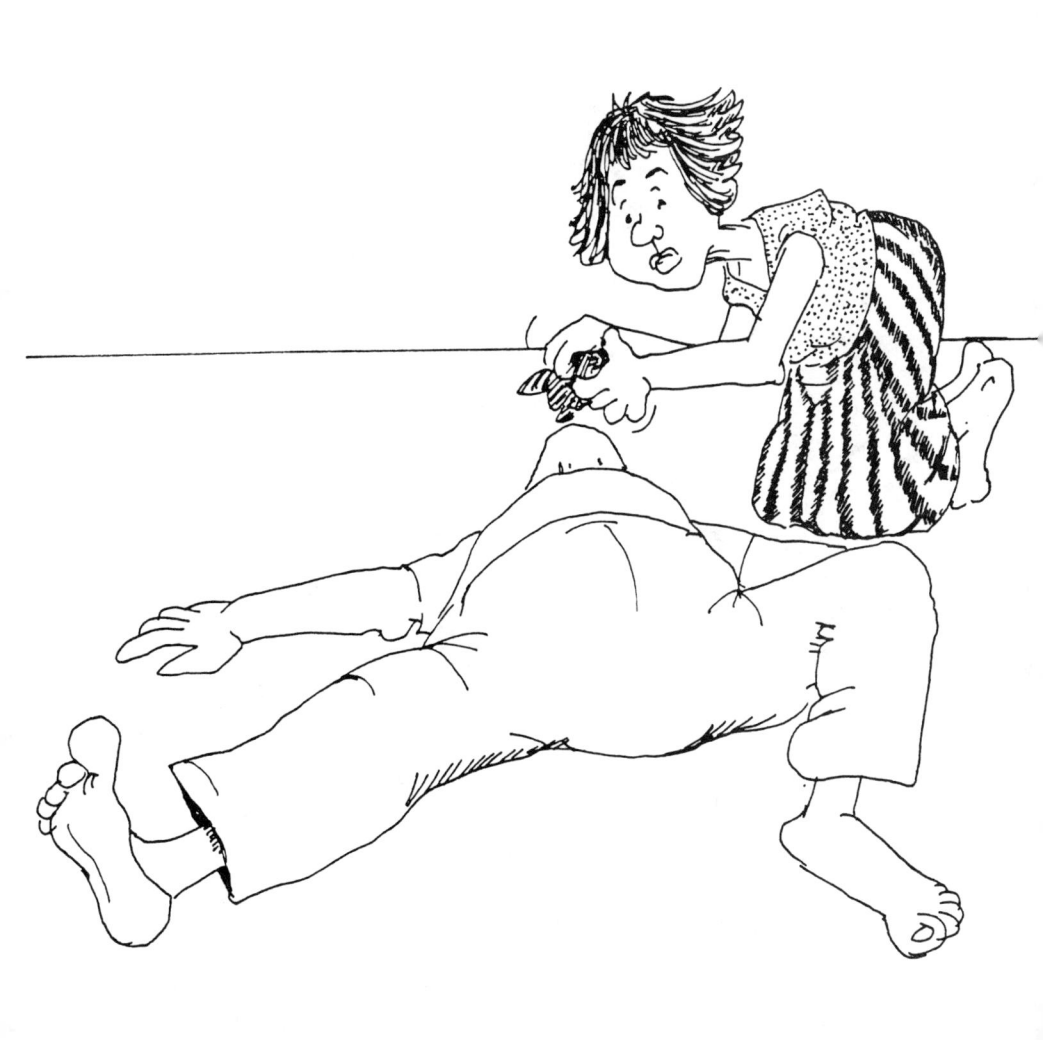

If a person faints, crush guava or soursop leaves and make him smell them.

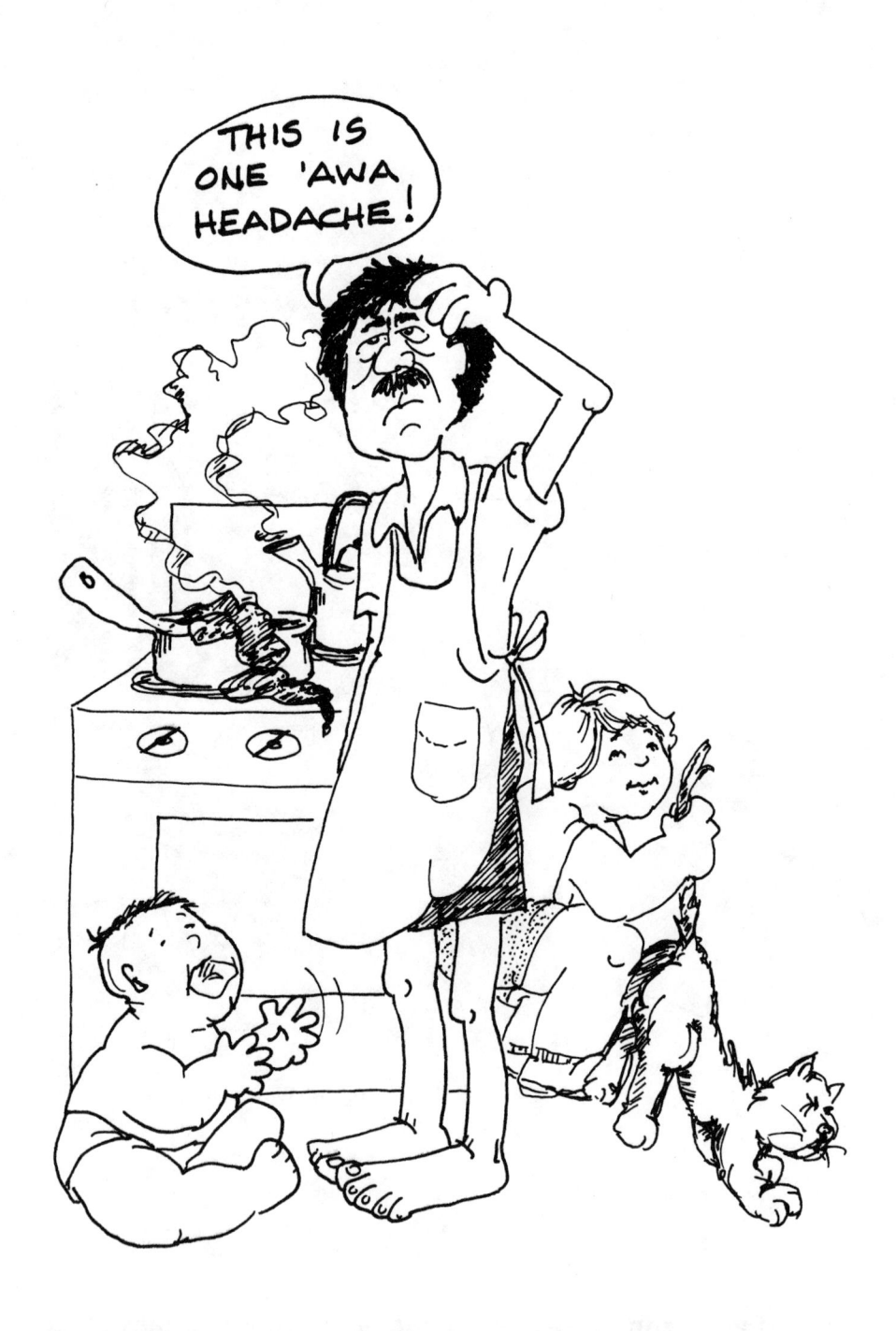

Chew 'awa root to relieve migrane headaches.

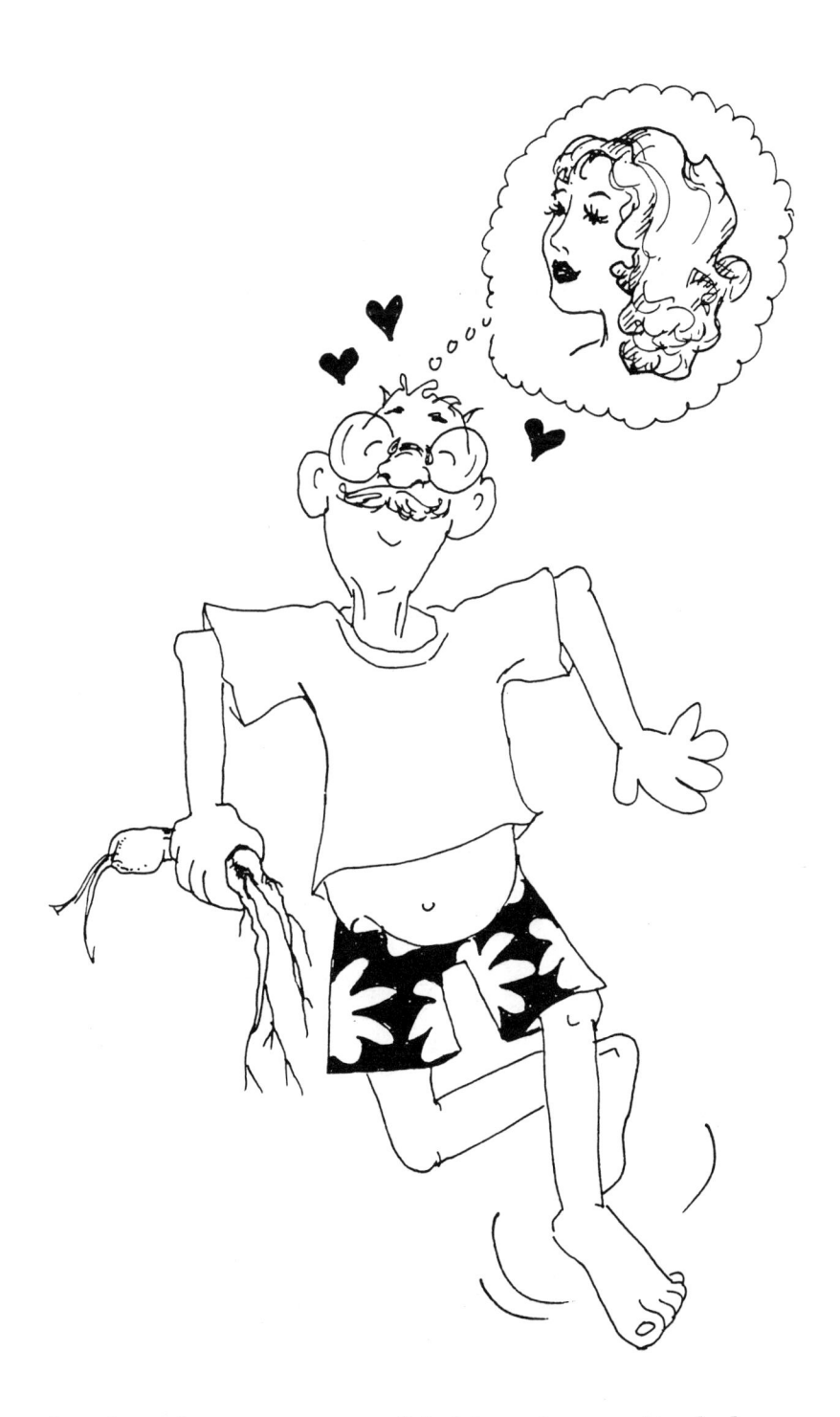

Chewing ginseng root or drinking ginseng tea helps a man maintain sexual potential and vitality.

A SHORT GLOSSARY OF REMEDIES

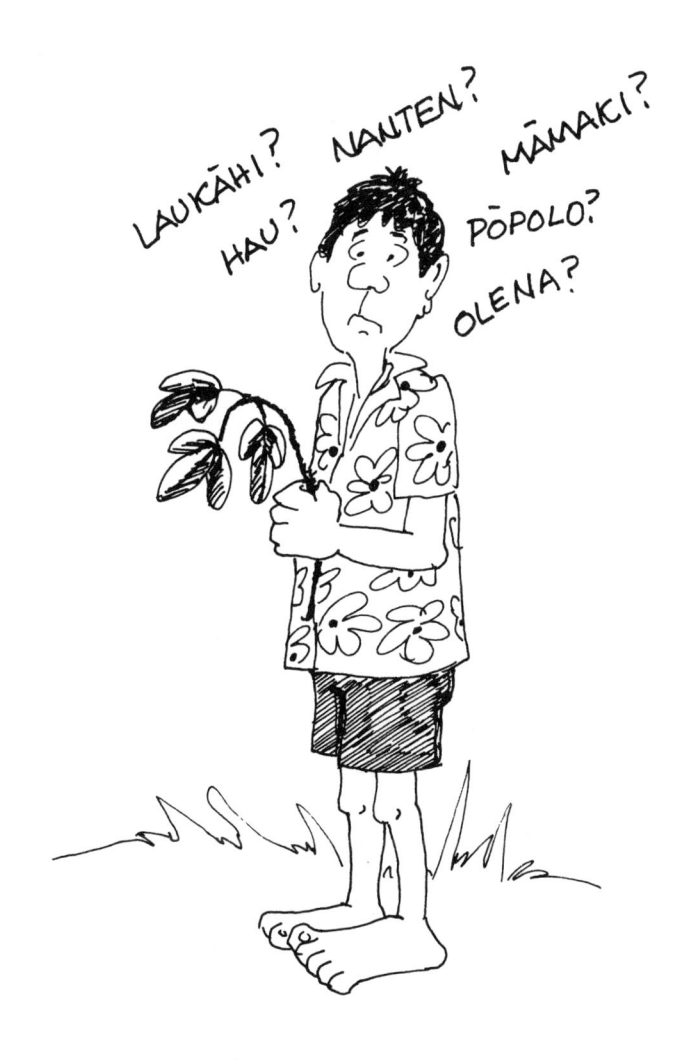

Aloe Vera

Throughout history, almost every culture has used aloe vera as a medicinal plant. A succulent plant with pale green leaves, aloe exudes a gel-like substance when it is cut. There are many medicinal varieties of aloe; however, in Hawai'i we are most familiar with the Mediterranean variety of aloe which is called panini 'awa 'awa in Hawaiian.

Aloe is used to treat burns, skin diseases, abrasions, and bruises. In addition, it is used as a laxative, as a medicine for kidney problems, and for stomach trouble.

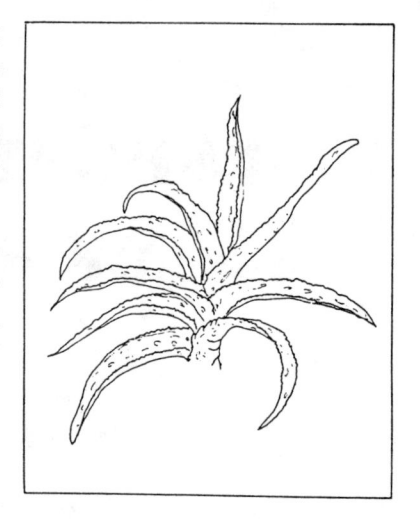

Arrowroot

see Pia

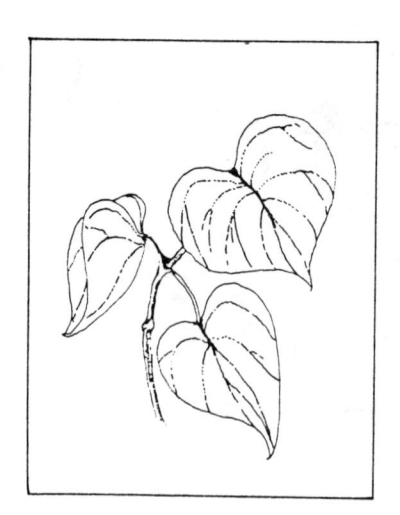

'Awa

The plant called 'awa in Hawai'i is known as kava in other parts of Polynesia. A member of the pepper family, it was brought to Hawai'i by early Polynesians and was a popular medicinal plant.

'Awa was drunk by Hawaiians as a sign of good will at ceremonies and festivities. It is used as medicine for numerous ailments including sore muscles, headaches, asthma, and insomnia. Because 'awa has a narcotic effect, it was formerly used as a sedative to calm the nerves or to set broken bones.

'Awapuhi kuahiwi

see Ginger, wild

'Awapuhi Pake:

see Ginger, Chinese

Banana

    Bananas were brought to Hawai'i by Polynesians. They were used mainly as food, but some varieties were used medicinally. The juice from banana blossoms served as a forerunner of vitamins for babies. The same juice was also used to treat sores of the mouth. Bananas were also prescribed to treat disorders of the stomach, asthma, and general weakness of the body.
    Bananas have been shown to have antibacterial properties. In addition, they contain a high level of potassium. Considered a neutralizer, bananas have been recommended for both diarrhea and constipation.

Breadfruit ('Ulu)

    'Ulu, or breadfruit, was brought to Hawai'i from Polynesia. It was a useful plant for its fruit was baked and eaten as a carbohydrate, the bark was used for tapa, and the trunk used for making poi boards. The sticky sap from the tree was used for medicinal purposes. It was frequently mixed with other plants and used for skin diseases and sores in the mouth.

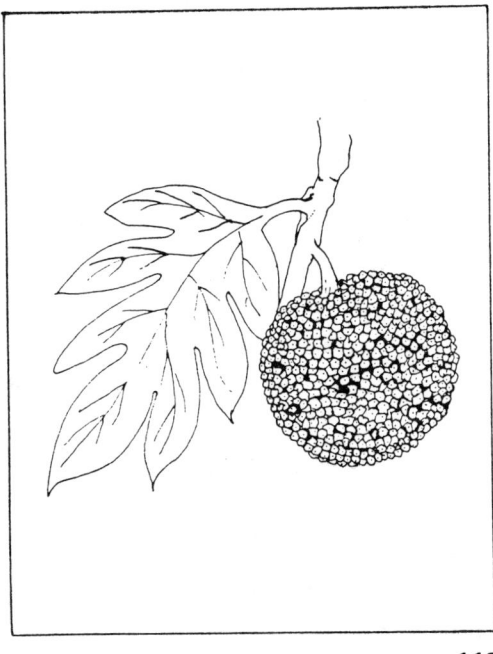

Eucalyptus

Eucalyptus trees were introduced to Hawai'i from Australia. There are many varieties of this tree which grows very tall and has fragrant, leathery leaves.

Eucalyptus leaves contain an oil, and have been used by various cultures to relieve asthma and congestion of the bronchial tubes. The leaves are also used as an antiseptic, and, boiled in water, they are used to treat aches and pains.

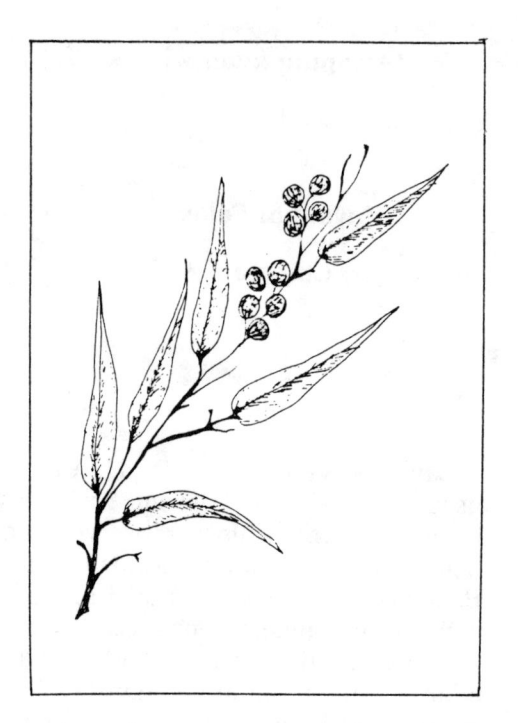

Garlic

Garlic has been popular in many countries as a folk remedy. Perhaps the reason for this is that garlic is strongly flavored, and in much folk wisdom, such foods are associated with strength. However, it is a fact that garlic does contain two antibacterial agents, allicin and alliin. Also, garlic has some essential oils in it which are said to dissolve cholesterol in humans. Throughout history, garlic has been used to treat numerous ailments ranging from indigestion to dandruff.

Ginger, Chinese ('Awapuhi Pake)

'Awapuhi Pake is the common ginger which we see in markets and grocery stores. It is also known as Jamaican ginger or Chinese ginger. The roots of the plant are used for flavoring foods and making ginger ale and candied ginger. But ginger root is also widely used as a medicinal plant by Orientals as well as Hawaiians. It has been used for fevers and colds, indigestion, and as an all-purpose energizer.

Ginger, Wild
('Awapuhi Kuahiwi)

'Awapuhi kuahiwi, or wild ginger, was brought to Hawai'i by the Polynesians. The underground stems of the plant were used as medicine by the ancient Hawaiians.

To prepare roots for medicinal purposes, the roots were washed and ground with a mortar and pestle. Water was added and the mixture was strained through fibers of makaloa (Hawaiian sedge). Sometimes the root was merely pounded and mixed with other plants and applied to sores and wounds.

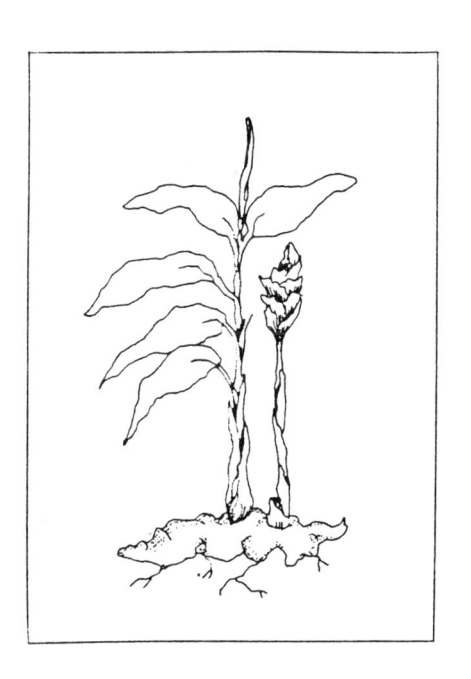

Ginseng

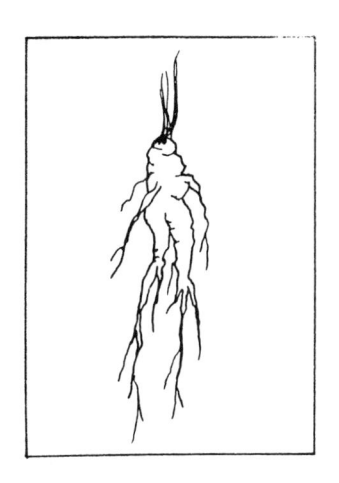

Ginseng, which is known as the "herb of eternal life," is thought to be an all purpose tonic and medicine. Many Orientals believe that regular use of ginseng prolongs life and prevents senility. It is also credited with being an aphrodisiac and helps to maintain sexual potency and virility in the human male. Ginseng is also believed to cure anemia, increase one's stamina, and prevent colds and sore throats. In addition, it has been prescribed for treatment of tuberculosis, nausea, diarrhea, gout, diabetes, jaundice, and insomnia.

Guava

The guava was brought to Hawai'i in the late 1700's by Don Marin, a Spaniard who introduced many tropical plants to the islands. The Hawaiians soon began to use it for medicinal purposes as well as for food.

Guava has been used to treat cuts, sprains, and other accidental injuries. Because it grows wild, it is often used for first aid treatment on injuries incurred on hikes. Leaf buds of the guava are used to make a tea to treat diarrhea and sore throats. Guava roots are used to treat bleeding from the bowels and intestines.

Hala (Pandanus)

It is not known whether the hala tree was growing in Hawai'i when the Polynesians arrived or whether they brought the tree with them. The tree was very useful for making hats, leis, and brushes.

Roots and flowers of the hala tree were used by Hawaiians as medicine. Aerial roots were pounded and mixed with other plants to make a tonic to strengthen the weak. Flowers were used to relieve constipation in children as well as adults.

Hau

Hau trees grow near the ocean. A kind of hibiscus, the plant is often crooked and gnarled. It has large, rounded leaves and flowers which change in color from yellow to dull red as the day progresses.

The hau tree was useful to Hawaiians for it provided them with wood for outriggers, bark for ropes, tapa, and bags, leaves for dishes, and bark and flowers for medicine. Medicinally, hau was used as a laxative, as a remedy for chest congestion, and as an aid in childbirth.

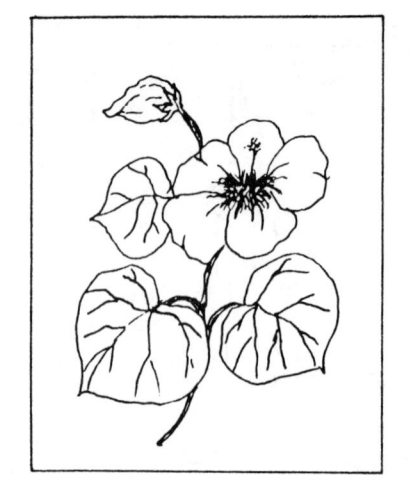

Honey

Honey has been used for thousands of years as a home remedy by people of many cultures. In recent years, the effectiveness of honey in treating various ailments has been documented in medicinal journals. Honey contains mainly fructose and glucose, but it also contains proteins, enzymes, small amounts of minerals and vitamins.

Honeysuckle

This fragrant vine is a popular folk medicine among Westerners as well as Orientals. Its therapeutic qualities include the ability to reduce inflammation. It has been used to treat fever, sore throat, mumps, laryngitis, boils, and skin sores.

Ilima

Ilima is generally known as a blossom for leis. It was used by ancient Hawaiians as a medicinal plant – as a mild laxative, as an aid to childbirth, as a general tonic, and as a treatment for colds and asthma.

Indian Mulberry:

see Noni

Kalo

see Taro

Kō

see Sugar Cane

Koali

see Morning glory

Kukui

The kukui nut tree was very useful to Hawaiians. Nuts were used for lamps and candles, for leis, and as a relish ('inamona). Medicinally, the bark, sap, and oil from the nuts are all used. Rich in oil, the nuts make a strong laxative and the sap from the stems is used to treat sores and ulcers of the skin.

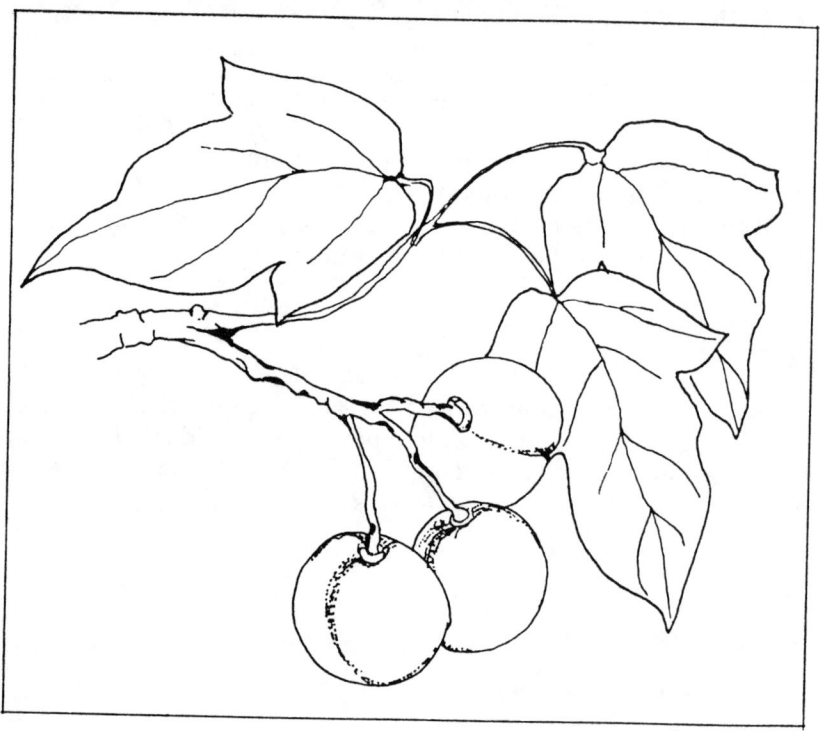

Lady Slipper ('Olepe)

A type of impatiens, this garden plant has a juicy stem and delicate flowers which range in color from white to pink and purple. All parts of the plant are used as medicine. It is used as a pain reliever for arthritis and rheumatism, as a treatment for coughs, and as a medicinal tea to flush the kidneys.

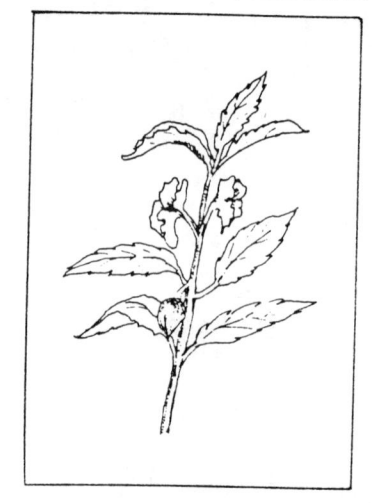

Lāpine

see Lemon Grass

Laukāhi

Laukāhi is a broadleaf weed which is common to lawns. This herb grows flat, without a stem, and its flowers are borne in spikes that rise above the flat leaves.

Laukāhi was a popular medicinal herb in ancient Hawai'i. It was used as a general tonic, as a laxative, and as a treatment for cuts and boils. Known as obako in Japanese, it is still used today as a medicinal plant by Hawaiians and Orientals.

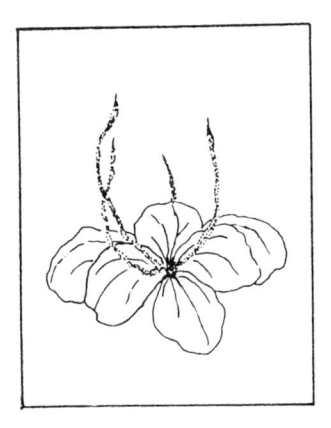

Lemon

The common lemon is universally recognized as a useful folk remedy for many ailments. In many cultures, lemon juice is used as an antiseptic, replacing rubbing alcohol or hydrogen peroxide.

Throughout the world, lemon juice is used as a tonic to keep the body functioning well and as a soother of frazzled nerves. It is also a universal remedy for sore throats and colds.

Lemon juice's active ingredients are vitamin C, citric acid, and some calcium, potassium, and bioflavonoids which keep capillaries resilient.

Lemon Grass (Lāpine)

Lemon grass is a fragrant oil grass which grows in tufts. The slender, rough-edged leaves produce a lemon scent when crushed.

Lemon grass is used for flavoring foods by Filipinos and Southeast Asians. In Hawai'i the leaves are frequently used in medicinal teas.

Limu (Seaweed)

Limu is a general name for plants which live under water (fresh, as well as salt) and algae and plants such as mosses. However, in general usage, limu means seaweed. There are several varieties of limu and they were utilized in many ways by the Hawaiians.

Limu kala (sargassum, or common yellow-brown seaweed) is frequently used as a ceremonial and medicinal plant. Readily available at the beach, it is often used to treat coral cuts. Other varieties of limu are used to relieve stomach aches, treat asthma, and general aches and pains. Research has shown that limu does have natural antibiotic properties.

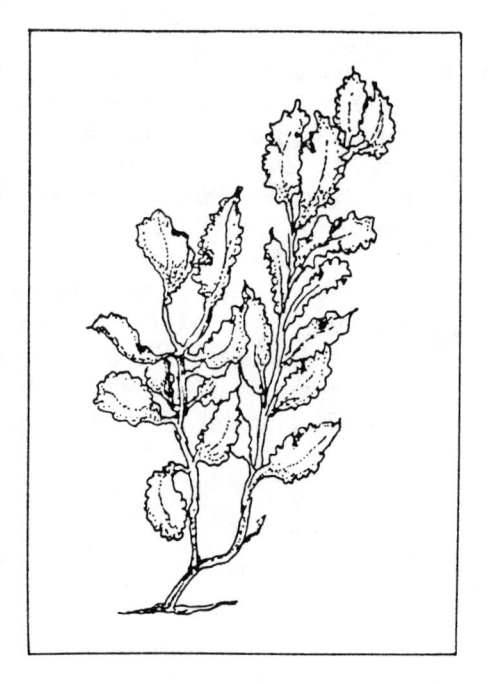

Māmaki

Māmaki, a native Hawaiian plant, is a tree-like shrub with berries similar to mulberries. Its bark was used to make tapa and clubs. Medicinally, māmaki seeds were used as a tonic to strengthen the body. Berries were used to heal sores and wounds, and māmaki tea is still prescribed today as a folk remedy for high blood pressure.

Morning Glory (Koali)

Two varieties of morning glory were used for medicine by Hawaiians. They are the common morning glory, koali 'awa, and the beach morning glory, or pōhuehue. Koali-'awa is a vine with heart-shaped leaves and blue flowers which turn pink as the day progresses. Pōhuehue grows along sandy beaches. It has smaller, rounded leaves and small, bell-shaped pink flowers.

The vines were used as a laxative. Roots, leaves, and flowers of koali 'awa were used for backaches and for healing broken bones. Pōhuehue was prescribed as an aid in childbirth.

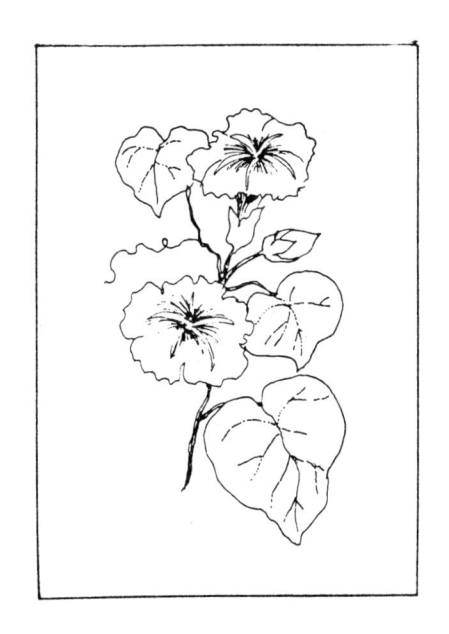

Mountain Apple

This handsome tree grows in valleys and cool areas of the islands. Bark, leaves, and fruit are of medicinal value. Mountain apple has been used to treat cuts, to build up the body after illnesses, and to heal sores of the mouth.

Moxa

This term refers to fiber obtained from the dried leaves of yomogi or wormwood. Japanese burn moxa on the body at specific vital spots (like acupuncture) to cure various ailments ranging from kidney and stomach ailments to bed wetting. The treatment used in this way is known as o-kyu or yaito. See also o-kyu.

Nandina

see Nanten

Nanten
(Nandina or Sacred Bamboo)

This attractive shrub is a favorite in Oriental gardens and is known as a good luck plant. Its rich, dark green leaves are said to be effective in reducing high fevers.

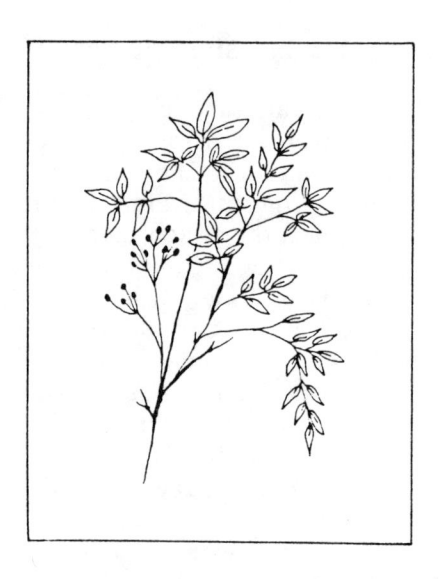

Noni (Indian Mulberry)

Noni is an evergreen shrub which grows in Asia, Australia, and Pacific islands. Brought to Hawai'i by Polynesians, it was very useful to ancient Hawaiians. The bark and roots of the plant were used to make dyes for tapa. The fruit resembles a small breadfruit and has a foul smell and unpleasant flavor. It was used to treat a number of ailments including diabetes, high blood pressure, heart trouble, and ukus (lice). The leaves of the plant were also used for medicinal purposes.

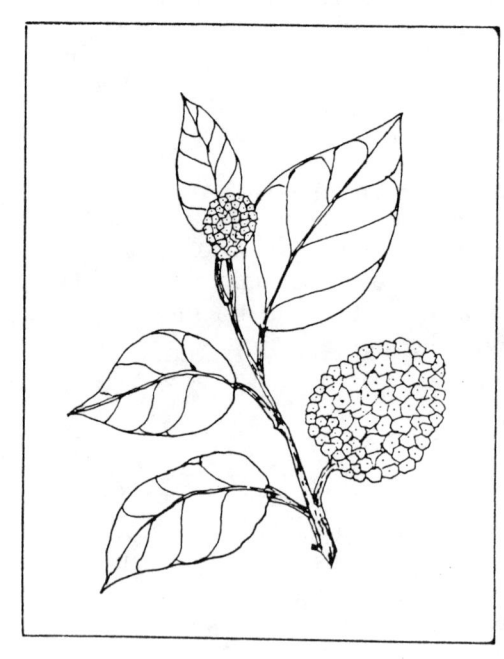

Obako

see Laukāhi

O-kyu

O-kyu, also called yaito, is a treatment for illnesses and for improving blood circulation by the application of heat to specific spots on the body. Moxa is placed on these spots (commonly along the spine or back of the knees) and burned with an incense stick. The principle of o-kyu rests on the theory of regulation of one's system by irritation and stimulation. O-kyu is also used on naughty children as punishment. See also moxa.

'Ōlena (Tumeric)

Like many other plants, 'ōlena was probably brought to the islands by migrating Polynesians. The plant was very useful as a dye plant. It is also of medicinal value. Mixed and pounded together with other plants, it can be used to gargle. The juice of the plant is also prescribed for earaches and, as a tea, it is said to relieve high blood pressure.

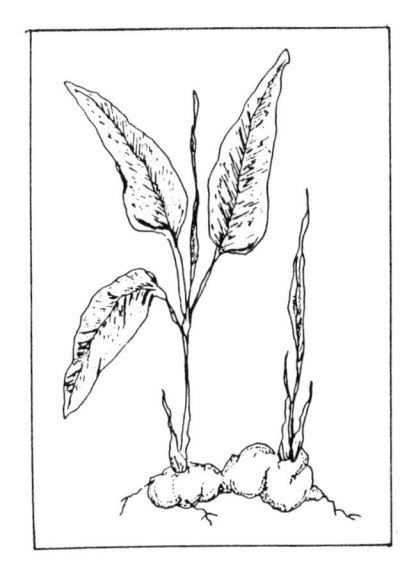

'Olepe

see Lady Slipper

Onion

The common yellow onion has been used by many cultures throughout history as a medicinal plant. Because it contains some sulphur, it is a natural disinfectant. Onions have been used as a remedy for colds and bronchial problems as well as for general maintenance of good health. It has also been said that onions are good for the heart. It may be taken as folk medicine by some, but researchers have proved that oils in both garlic and onion help to reduce cholesterol levels in the blood.

Externally, onions or onion juice has been used to soothe insect bites and stings and to remove skin blemishes. Onions were brought to Hawai'i by Europeans, and Hawaiians soon adopted them for medicinal use. Early Hawaiians used onion juice to cure eye and ear problems.

Pandanus

see Hala

Papaya

Papaya has long been used in the tropical world as a medicinal plant. It is not known when papaya was introduced to Hawai'i, but it is thought it was introduced to the islands by way of Asia and Polynesia sometime before the arrival of the first Europeans. Nearly all parts of the plant have medicinal value. The sap from the fruit has been used to treat skin diseases and the leaves have been used to treat insect bites. Seeds of the fruit have been used to treat a variety of ailments ranging from earaches to pinworms. Although not yet proven, it is said that papaya seed may be an effective treatment for cancer.

Pia (Arrowroot)

Pia, or Polynesian arrowroot, is a plant known throughout the Pacific and tropical parts of Asia, Africa, and Australia. It was probably brought to Hawai'i by people who came from Asia. Hawaiians grated the tubers and removed a starch from them. The starch obtained from pia is similar to cornstarch, and can be used as a thickening agent. The tubers were also used medicinally to treat diarrhea and dysentery.

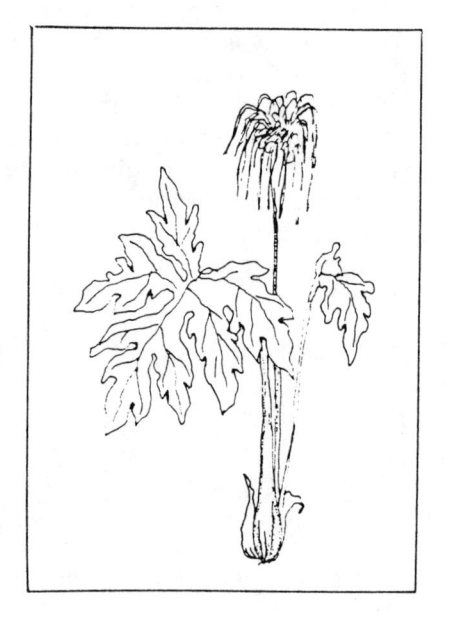

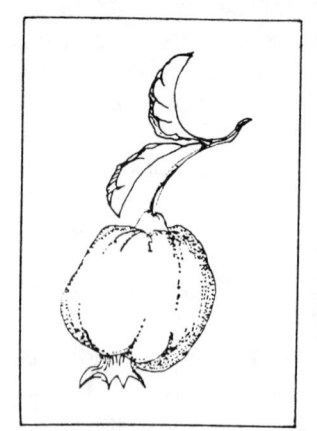

Pomegranate

This is an attractive shrub with leathery-skinned fruit full of transparent, juicy seeds. The acid fruit is used by Orientals to treat stomach aches and sore throats.

Pomelo

Also known as jabon, locally, this is a kind of grapefruit. The skin is thick and leathery, and the fruit is of a coarse texture. Pomelo skin and leaves are used medicinally for colds and sore throats.

Pōpolo

A common weed in Hawai'i, pōpolo has been called "the foundation of Hawaiian pharmacy." An important medicinal plant in Hawaiian culture, it is used to treat cuts, wounds, and skin eruptions as well as to treat colds and ailments of the bronchial and digestive tracts. Ancient Hawaiians regarded pōpolo as an embodiment of the god Kane, and it is referred to as Kane-pōpolo.

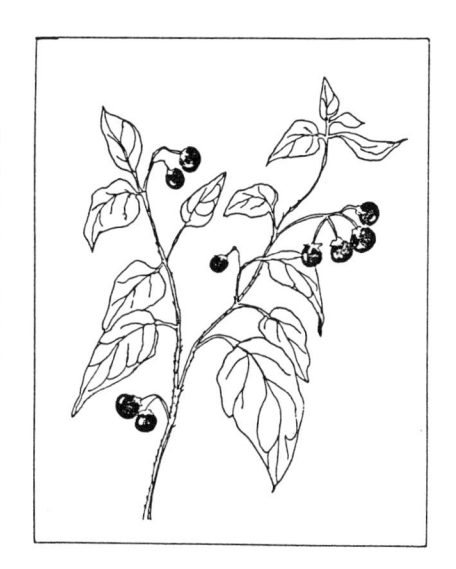

Poppy

see Pua-Kala

Pua-Kala
(Beach or Prickly Poppy)

A Hawaiian variety of the common poppy, this plant grows near the seacoast. It has a coarse, prickly stem and leaves and delicate white flowers. Like other poppy plants, pua-kala contains a mild narcotic in its juice. It was used by Hawaiians to relieve minor pains such as toothaches.

Sacred Bamboo

see Nanten

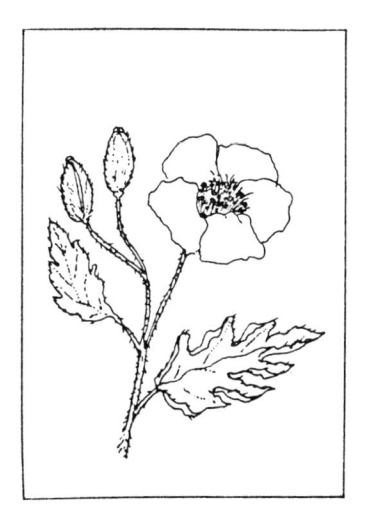

Salt and Sea Water

Throughout history, salt has been considered sacred. It preserves things and does not rot, and therefore it has become a symbol of eternity. Because of its curative qualities, countless superstitions and charms are connected with salt. It is present in almost all cultures as a folk remedy for various ailments.

The Hawaiians, like other people, relied on salt and the sea as a remedy for many illnesses. It was used as an antiseptic to cleanse wounds. It was also used as a remedy for stomach ailments, sore throats, aches and pains, and sinus problems. Salt was also used in rituals to remove evil spirits from the body.

Seaweed

see Limu

Soups

There is no proven cure for the common cold, but chicken soup ranks high on the list of cold cures. There is now scientific evidence that hot chicken soup clears mucus from the nostrils, and hence, lessens the time viruses are in contact with the nose. While researchers suspect that there is a chemical ingredient in chicken soup and not just the vapors that cure a cold, they are not certain of what does the trick.

Almost every ethnic group has its own version of a nourishing soup. Chicken, beef shanks, pork, and even chicken feet are used as the basis of these soups. The Japanese swear by miso soup, while Koreans recommend seaweed soup. With slight variation of ingredients, these soups provide nourishing and loving substance to the sick and convalescing.

Spanish Needle

A common weed in Hawai'i, this plant bears flowers with spiny needles. This plant has long been used in Hawai'i as a tea to maintain general health and to lower high blood pressure.

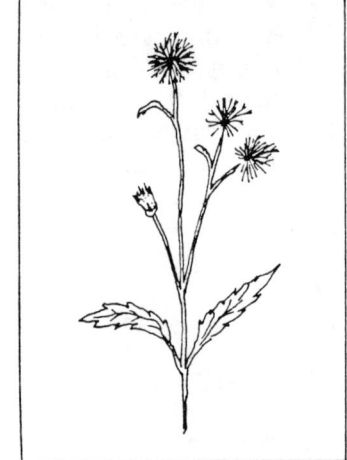

Sugar Cane (Kō)

Sugar cane was brought to the islands by the Polynesians. While young shoots of cane were used to treat cuts and wounds, cane was used mainly as a sweetening agent with other medicinal plants. A stalk of cane was cut and the tough outer layer removed. The sweet sap was then squeezed out and mixed with other ingredients.

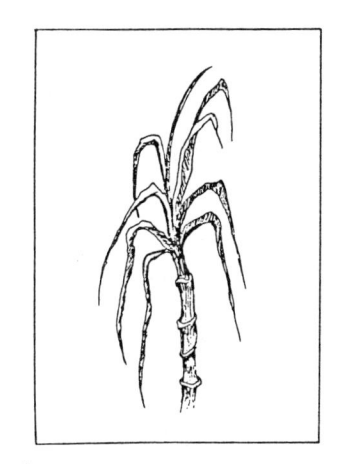

Sweet Potato ('Uala)

This plant was problably brought to Hawai'i by migrating Polynesians. The ancient Hawaiians used the tuber and greens as food. In addition, fermented tubers were used as a kind of beer called 'uala 'awa 'awa.

Various parts of the plant were used in medicinal treatment. The tuber, mixed with water and other plants, was used to treat asthma, constipation, and vomiting. Vines and leaves were used to induce vomiting. The vines were also worn around the neck by nursing mothers to make milk flow after childbirth.

Taro (Kalo)

There were many varieties of taro in ancient Hawai'i, all of which had crystals which irritate the mouth if eaten uncooked. Some varieties of taro had fewer crystals, and these were used for medicinal purposes. To prepare taro for medicine, the uncooked corm was scraped with the edge of a knife and the pulp or juice was swallowed. For a band-aid, Hawaiians tied a raw slice of taro on the wound. The astringent quality of the crystals in taro helped to stop bleeding. The raw stem of the taro plant was used to treat cuts and insect bites.

Poi, which is made out of steamed taro corms, has been praised as a health food. A carbohydrate, it is low in fat, and contains vitamin B, calcium and phosphorus. It is easily digested and is often recommended as a first solid food for infants in Hawai'i. In addition, poi can be used as a poultice on infected sores.

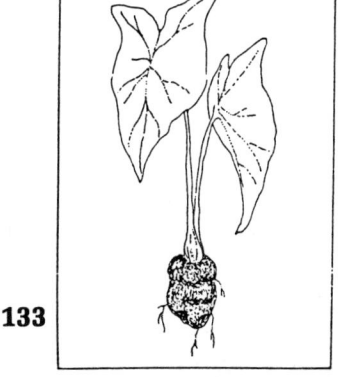

Ti (Kī)

The common ti plant was a most useful plant among Hawaiians. It was used for cooking and serving food, for dress and shelter, as an important ceremonial plant, and as medicine.

Ti leaves are believed by Hawaiians to have protective qualities, protecting one from evil spirits. Ti was also used to exorcise evil from the body. Pounded ti root was mixed with other plants to relieve asthma and young shoots were said to treat coughs. Ti leaves were frequently used to treat fevers and to remove poisons from the body.

Tumeric

see 'Olena

'Uala

see Sweet Potato

'Uhaloa
(Waltheria Americana)

This weed is used medicinally in many cultures. It is said that the roots have the same effect as aspirin in relieving pain. The roots, leaves, and flowers are used to treat asthma, sore throats, and colds.

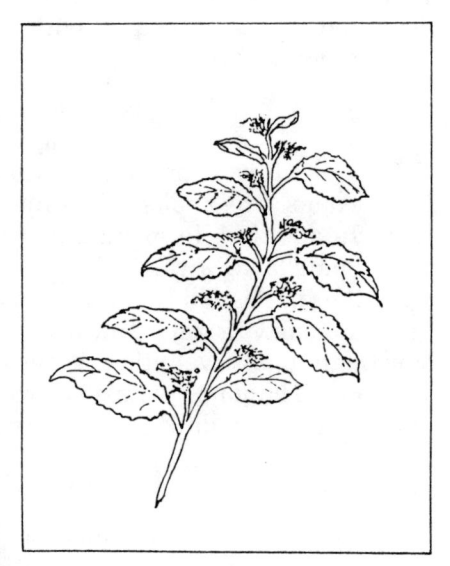

'Ulu

see Breadfruit

Ume

Also known as umeboshi, this pickled plum is indispensable to the Japanese. It is frequently eaten at the end of a meal, but it is also used as a treatment for colds and indigestion.

Urine

Body wastes have often been creditied with magical powers by primitive men. While these powers may or may not be true, it is a scientific fact that urine does have antiseptic powers as it contains both ammonia and salt. In emergency situations, urine has been used as an antiseptic. And urea, a component of urine, is used commercially as a healing agent in cosmetics and medications.

Yaito

see O-Kyu

Yomogi (Mugwort)

A member of the daisy family, this herb has greyish-green, fuzzy stems and leaves and small yellowish-green flowers. It is used by many nationalities as a medicinal tonic. The Japanese use leaves of yomogi for moxa, a soft fuzz used to burn the skin at certain points to cure a number of ailments.

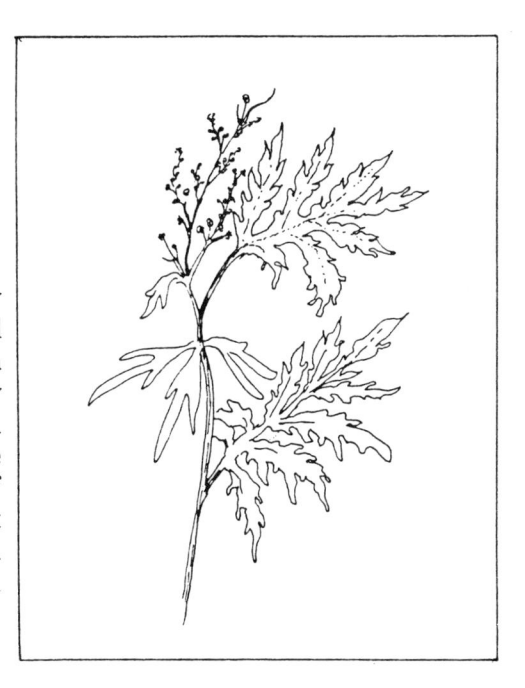

Readings

Gutmanis, June. *Kahuna La'au Lapa'au: The Practice of Hawaiian Herbal Medicine.* Honolulu: Island Heritage, 1979.

Handy, E. S. Craighill and Elizabeth Green. *Native Planters in Old Hawai'i: Their Life, Lore, and Environment.* Bishop Museum Bulletin 233. Honolulu: Bishop Museum Press, 1972.

Handy, E. S. Craighill with Mary Kawena Pukui and Katherine Livermore. *Outline of Hawaiian Physical Therapeutics.* Bishop Museum Bulletin 126. Honolulu: Bishop Museum Press, 1934.

Hyatt, Richard. *Chinese Herbal Medicine: An Ancient Art and Modern Healing Practice.* New York: Thorsons, 1984.

Joya, Mock. *Things Japanese.* Tokyo: Tokyo News Service, 1960.

Kaaiakamanu, D.M. and J. K. Akina. *Hawaiian Herbs of Medicinal Value.* Territorial Board of Health Bulletin, 1922, reprint, Honolulu: Pacific Book House.

Kamakau, Samuel Manaiakalani. *Ka Po'e Kahiko: The People of Old.* Honolulu: Bishop Museum Press, 1964.

Kordel, Lelord. *Natural Folk Remedies.* New York: Putnam, 1974.

Krauss, Beatrice H. *Ethnobotany of Hawai'i.* Honolulu, University of Hawai'i Department of Botany, n.d.

Krauss, Beatrice H. *Native Plants Used as Medicine in Hawai'i.* Honolulu: 1979 (pamphlet).

Le Strange, Richard. *A History of Herbal Plants.* New York: Arco, 1977.

Leung, Albert Y. *Chinese Herbal Remedies.* New York: Universe Books, 1984.

McBride, L.R. *Practical Folk Medicine of Hawai'i.* Hilo: Petroglyph Press, 1975.

Neal, Marie C. *In Gardens of Hawai'i.* Honolulu: Bishop Museum Press, 1965.

Rinzler, Carol Ann. *Dictionary of Medical Folklore.* New York: Crowell, 1979.

Tan, Terry. *Cooking with Chinese Herbs.* Singapore Times Books International, 1983.

Thomson, Robert. *The Grosset Encyclopedia of Natural Medicine.* New York: Grosset and Dunlap, 1980.

Weiner, Michael A. *Weiner's Herbal The Guide to Herb Medicine.* New York: Stein and Day, 1980.